AF790312

HEALTH SYSTEMS RESEARCH

Edited by W. van Eimeren

This book has been realized through the close collaboration between Battelle Medical Technology and Policy Research Center, Washington DC, Ciba-Geigy Basel and Interdisciplinary Research Centre for Public Health, St. Gallen

B. R. Luce A. Elixhauser

Standards for the Socioeconomic Evaluation of Health Care Services

Edited by A. J. Culyer

Postscript by B. Horisberger

With 17 Figures and 20 Tables

Springer-Verlag
Berlin Heidelberg New York
London Paris Tokyo Hong Kong

Bryan R. Luce, Ph. D.
Anne Elixhauser, Ph. D.
Battelle
Medical Technology and Policy Research Center
370 L'Enfant Promenade, S. W., Suite 900
Washington DC 20024-2115, USA

A. J. Culyer, Prof.
Department of Economics and Related Studies
University of York,
Heslington, York, England, Yol 5DD

Bruno Horisberger, M.D.
Interdisciplinary Research Centre
for Public Health
Rorschacher Straße 103c
CH-9007 St. Gallen
Switzerland

ISBN-13:978-3-642-75492-0 e-ISBN-13:978-3-642-75490-6
DOI: 10.1007/978-3-642-75490-6

This work is subject to copyright. All rights are reserved, whether the whole or part of the material is concerned, specifically the rights of translation, reprinting, reuse of illustration, recitation, broadcasting, reproduction on microfilms or in other ways, and storage in data banks. Duplication of this publication or parts thereof is only permitted under the provisions of the German Copyright Law of September 9, 1965, in its current version, and a copyright feet must always be paid. Violations fall under the prosecution act of the German Copyright Law.

© Springer-Verlag Berlin Heidelberg 1990
Softcover reprint of the hardcover 1st edition 1990

The use of general descriptive names, trade marks, etc. in this publication, even if the former are not especially identified, is not to be taken as a sign that such names, as understood by the Trade marks and Merchandise Marks Act, may accordingly be used by anyone.

Product Liability: The publisher can give no guarantee for information about drug dosage and application thereof contained in this book. In every individual case the respective user must check its a accuracy by consulting other pharmaceutical literature.

2119/3140/543210 – Printed on acid-free paper

Foreword

Over the past decades, health care delivery – once characterized by clearly defined relationships between medical professionals, regulators, and industry – has become much more complex. Traditional roles and relationships are changing and new decision-makers are entering the scene. They bring into the discussion the need for cost containment and the changing perceptions of the public with regard to the risks and benefits of health care outcomes. As benefits of medical care are increasingly questioned and as scepticism and fear of advanced technologies are demonstrated by a growing body of people, decision making must move beyond medical concerns to encompass economic, political, and sociological considerations.

This evolution has also affected the pharmaceutical industry. Public perception of responsibility for product safety is no longer limited to regulators and physicians. Manufacturers, previously unencumbered by social policies, governmental preoccupations, or public expectations, are now held accountable for product safety. As a certain amount of risk acceptance is, however, a prerequisite for the further development of health care goods, it has to be carefully balanced against society's demand for safety. To weigh risks against benefits, to define acceptable risk, and to exclude what no longer falls within this category remain perpetual challenges.

Accordingly, health care outcomes have to be assessed not only from a clinical point of view, but also from an economic and societal perspective. The assessment of drug risks and benefits has become an important political issue world-wide. Attention focuses on interdisciplinary research and management approaches in the areas of drug risk and benefit identification, quantification, assessment, and communication. Annual meetings at Wolfsberg, Switzerland, serve as a platform for international exchange on health care issues, e.g., cost sharing and technology assessment.

The first Wolfsberg Conference in 1987 strengthened this tradition, focusing on the socioeconomic evaluation of drug therapy (Conference Proceedings: "Socioeconomic Evaluation of Drug Therapy", 1988). It was recognized that it is no longer sufficient for pharmaceutical preparations to demonstrate quality, efficacy, and safety. Additional parameters, such as the evidence of cost-benefit and quality of life, have to be investigated. It will be mandatory to show that the benefits of a medicine – in terms of savings in other health care resources or in improved health – justify the costs, and that the product fulfills the basic efficiency requirement of "value for money."

The second Wolfsberg meeting in 1988 responded to the intensified public debate on drug risks, benefits, and safety (Conference Proceedings: "The Perception and Management of Drug Safety Risks," 1989). The focus was shifted from socioeconomic evaluation of drug therapy to integrating public perception and concern with drug risks. The understanding and management of drug safety is – in spite of improved drug surveillance activities – beset by doubts, disagreements, and disputes. Public disputes over risks are brought to court when individuals seek compensation for health problems attributed to a pharmaceutical product. Conflict occurs over the significance of risk, the adequacy of evidence, the methodologies used to evaluate and measure risk, the standards that guide regulation, and the optimal means of communicating risk information to the public.

The conference revealed that by addressing the public's questions and concerns, the pharmaceutical industry can significantly contribute to slowing down the negative cycle and initiating a positive one, marked by social responsibility, open communication, and trust. The definition of key drug-safety issues and a sense of how these issues might be addressed cooperatively led to the creation of the "RAD-AR" initiative. RAD-AR (Risk/Benefit Assessment of Drugs – Analysis and Response) represents a collaborative effort to improve drug safety through better assessment and communication of drug benefits and risks. RAD-AR member companies expressed their commitment to "improve dramatically the knowledge and understanding of both the risks and benefits of pharmaceuticals. Such improved knowledge and understanding is essential to facilitate better individual and collective decision-making regarding the availability and use of pharmaceuticals." RAD-AR projects currently fall into two main areas. In the area of assessment and appraisal, national and international interest groups are working to make existing pharmacoepidemiological data more useful and develop systems for collecting new data to increase quality of information on drug benefits and risks. In the area of perception and communication, the groups are working to understand better the processing of drug safety information and risk communication. The "Standards for Socioeconomic Evaluation of Health Care Products and Services" is the third publication following the 1987 and 1988 Wolfsberg proceedings. It goes beyond solely examining risk and benefits, by putting the two into a balanced perspective. Thus, the manual seeks to close the gap between drug risk and benefit issues by providing a methodology through which common standards for both parts of the drug safety balance can be equally applied. For decision-makers the standards will serve as a guide for systematic evaluation and will allow them to appropriately interpret and apply the results from socioeconomic evaluation.

Looking into the future, the mission of RAD-AR will further expand to progressively integrate the various societal perspectives, continuously responding to the need of balancing drug risk and benefits. This requires an ongoing exchange on new developments in benefit/risk assessment, appraisal, perception, communication, and management. A consensus has to be reached on future plans of action by regulatory authorities, pharmaceutical manufacturers, academic leaders, physicians, pharmacists, and interested media representatives.

W. P. von Wartburg

Contents

Editor's Introduction
A. J. Culyer XV

Socioeconomic Evaluations: an Executive Summary
A. J. Culyer, B. Luce and A. Elixhauser 1

Part I: Guidelines for the Evaluator

1 Introduction to Socioeconomic Evaluations 15
1.1 Introduction 15
1.2 Brief History of Socioeconomic Evaluations 15
1.3 Compromises and Choices in Socioeconomic Evaluation 15
1.4 Why Socioeconomic Evaluations Are Performed 19
1.5 Organization of the Text 19

2 Concepts in Socioeconomic Evaluation 21
2.1 Introduction 21
2.2 Generating Socioeconomic Hypotheses 22
2.3 Socioeconomic Concepts 23
2.3.1 Costs 23
2.3.2 Consequences 25
2.3.3 Marginal Analysis 26
2.4 Discounting and the Dimension of Time 28
2.5 Conclusion 29

3 Types of Socioeconomic Evaluation 30
3.1 Introduction 30
3.2 Types of Socioeconomic Evaluation 30
3.2.1 Cost-Benefit Analysis 32
3.2.2 Cost-Utility Analysis 35

3.2.3 Cost-Effectiveness Analysis . . . 37
3.2.4 Cost-Minimization Analysis . . . 38
3.2.5 Cost of Illness Studies . . . 39
3.2.6 Quality of Life Studies . . . 40
3.2.7 Budgetary Analysis . . . 42
3.3 Conclusion . . . 42

4 *Framework of the Evaluation* . . . 44
4.1 Introduction . . . 44
4.2 Defining the Research Question . . . 44
4.3 The Perspective . . . 45
4.3.1 The Perspective of Society . . . 45
4.3.2 The Perspective of the Third Party Payer . . . 47
4.3.3 The Perspective of the Health Care Provider . . . 48
4.3.4 The Patient's Perspective . . . 48
4.3.5 Perspective: An Overview . . . 49
4.4 The Alternatives . . . 49
4.4.1 The Research Question: An Overview . . . 51
4.5 Pathways of Clinical Management . . . 51
4.6 Conclusion . . . 55

5 *Assessing Costs* . . . 56
5.1 Introduction . . . 56
5.2 Types of Costs . . . 57
5.3 Determinants of the Types of Costs To Incorporate into Analysis . . . 61
5.3.1 Type of Analysis . . . 61
5.3.2 Alternatives . . . 61
5.3.3 Perspective . . . 61
5.4 Process of Identifying Costs . . . 62
5.5 Assigning Monetary Values to Resources . . . 63
5.6 Monetary Valuation of Consequences . . . 64
5.7 Specific Types of Costs . . . 64
5.8 Common Problems in Estimating Costs . . . 65
5.9 Conclusion . . . 66

6 *Assessing Consequences* . . . 68
6.1 Introduction . . . 68
6.2 Types of Consequences . . . 68
6.2.1 Clinical Consequences . . . 68
6.2.2 Psychosocial Consequences . . . 70

6.2.3 Economic Consequences 71
6.3 Determinants of Which Consequences Are Included in an Analysis . 72
6.3.1 Type of Study 72
6.3.2 Research Question 73
6.3.3 Perspective 73
6.4 Medication Compliance 74
6.5 Conclusion 74

7 Adjusting Costs and Consequences 77
7.1 Introduction 77
7.2 Discounting 77
7.3 Sensitivity Analysis 80
7.4 Conclusion 82

8 Issues in Study Design 83
8.1 Introduction 83
8.2 Measurement of Consequences 83
8.3 Dimensions of Study Design 85
8.3.1 Prospective Studies 85
8.3.2 Pre-test Post-test Design 87
8.3.3 Quasi-experimental Designs 88
8.3.4 Variations on Prospective Studies 89
8.3.5 Retrospective Studies 90
8.4 Modeling 91
8.5 Conclusion 93

9 How To Assess a Socioeconomic Evaluation 94
9.1 Introduction 94
9.2 Guide for Evaluating Socioeconomic Evaluations 94
9.3 Case Study 1 98
9.4 Case Study 2 102

Part II: Technical Aspects

10 Quality of Life Assessment in Socioeconomic Evaluations 109
10.1 Definition of Quality of Life 109
10.2 Importance of Quality of Life Assessment 111
10.3 Measurement of Quality of Life 112
10.4 Conclusion 113

10.5 Examples of Quality of Life Scale Items . . . 113
10.5.1 Social Functioning . . . 114
10.5.2 Physical Functioning . . . 114
10.5.3 Emotional Functioning . . . 114
10.5.4 Intellectual Functioning . . . 115
10.5.5 General Well-being . . . 115
Further Reading . . . 115

11 Decision Analysis . . . 117
11.1 Definition of Decision Analysis . . . 117
11.2 Bayes' Theorem . . . 117
11.3 Decision Trees . . . 118
11.4 Sensitivity Analysis . . . 120
11.5 Markov Processes . . . 121
11.6 Conclusion . . . 122
Further Reading . . . 123

12 Utility Analysis in Socioeconomic Evaluation . . . 124
12.1 Cost-Utility Analysis and Health State Utilities . . . 124
12.2 Methods for Assessing Health State Utilities . . . 125
Further Reading . . . 126

13 Background on Statistics: Fundamental Concepts . . . 127
13.1 Measures of Central Tendency and Dispersion . . . 127
13.2 Hypothesis Testing . . . 128
13.3 Statistical Significance . . . 128
13.4 Type I and Type II Error . . . 129
13.5 Power . . . 130
13.6 Sample Size . . . 130
Further Reading . . . 133

14 Basic Analytica Techniques . . . 134
14.1 Levels of Measurement . . . 134
14.2 Parametric and Nonparametric Tests . . . 135
14.3 Commonly Used Statistical Techniques . . . 135
14.3.1 t-Test . . . 135
14.3.2 Analysis of Variance . . . 136
14.3.3 Chi-square Test . . . 136
14.3.4 Correlation Analysis . . . 140
14.3.5 Ordinary Least Squares Regression . . . 141

Glossary 144

References 159

Postscript: Successful Socioeconomic Evaluation of Health Care Services
B. HORISBERGER 163

Curriculum Vitae of Authors 179

Subject Index 181

Acknowledgments

This book would not have been possible without the insight, support, and labor of several individuals. Jorge Wernli and Peter Lauper at Ciba-Geigy conceived of the idea of creating a book about the application of the socioeconomic evaluation of drug therapies.

They envisioned a clear and uncomplicated discussion of socioeconomic evaluation methods in accordance with the most current theory and practice. Under their direction, this project grew and developed into a broader and more comprehensive text, intended to meet the needs of evaluators in pharmaceutical companies and of health care decision-makers.

Dr. Burton Weisbrod of the University of Wisconsin contributed his thoughtful ideas throughout the project. He provided insight and creativity, both in organizing the text and in expressing these concepts clearly and accurately.

Finally, the generous support of Ciba-Geigy is gratefully acknowledged.

Editor's Introduction

A. J. CULYER

This clearly structured, authoritative manual prepared by Bryan R. Luce and Anne Elixhauser from the Battelle Medical Technology and Policy Research Center in Washington, DC, United States, is written for those who read and use socioeconomic evaluations of medications. It is intended to enable them to be better *commissioners* of socioeconomic evaluations, to be more effective *partners* in the conduct of such studies, and to be more critical *assessors* of the quality of the evaluations that are provided by research teams.

The authoritative account which follows is commended as an up-to-date briefing on the fast-changing technology of socioeconomic evaluation. Socioeconomic evaluation is quintessentially multidisciplinary and requires, if it is to be done well, the active collaboration of medical scientists, social scientists, and health service policymakers and managers. For these reasons it is essential that accessible accounts of its methods, achievements, and pitfalls become periodically available beyond the arcane circle of the *cognoscenti*. It is with this in mind that the present text has been prepared.

Socioeconomic Evaluations: an Executive Summary

A. J. CULYER, B. LUCE and A. ELIXHAUSER

In the past, decisions about the use of health care technologies were based solely on the clinical safety and efficacy of the technology. Upwardly spiraling medical costs as well as the unique burden associated with managing chronic disease have sensitized health care decision-makers in both the private and the public sector to the problems of scarce resources and multiple competing interventions. These problems have pressed decision-makers to examine additional criteria in deciding whether and when to use and pay for a particular technology.

The techniques of socioeconomic evaluation have progressed rapidly, and continue to progress. There is now widespread agreement that such multidisciplinary evaluation is an important aid to decision-makers. Although numerous evaluations of technologies have been reported, the quality of the research has been variable and there is the danger that the increasing sophistication of evaluative technology distances analysts from decision-makers. Consequently there is now a well-perceived need among decision-makers for guidance as to the principles and methods available and for help in interpreting studies, judging their quality, and determining their applicability to particular settings.

> Health care decision-makers need guidance in commissioning, interpreting, and applying the results of socioeconomic evaluations.

This book attempts to provide just such a guide. Its illustrations are from the technologies of medication, but its lessons are much broader than that. The main text is divided into two parts. Part I ("Guidelines for the Evaluator") is a nontechnical introduction to the principles and methods with copious practical illustrations. Part II ("Technical Aspects") picks up some of the principal methods currently in use, discusses them in greater depth, and provides further reading for those wishing to acquire a more fundamental grasp. This introduction provides an overview of what is in the rest of the book.

Definition of Socioeconomic Evaluations

Socioeconomic evaluations use research methods based on the social sciences, primarily economics and psychology. They are methods which enumerate the costs and consequences associated with medical products and services, such as medications.

Socioeconomic evaluations enumerate the costs and/or consequences associated with medical products and services.

Costs are the monetary valuations of resource inputs required to produce a health outcome. *Consequences* are the monetary and nonmonetary outcomes of applying a particular intervention. It is vital to recognize that socioeconomic evaluations are grounded in the clinical efficacy of the interventions which they evaluate. The clinical effects of a medications must be clearly understood (including any uncertainty about the effects) before the relevant socioeconomic hypotheses can be generated.

It is helpful to visualize two streams of events pertaining to each medical intervention. The first is the medical stream. In this stream, a patient arrives at a physician's office, receives treatment, and is cured or not. Paralleling this stream is the socioeconomic stream of events. Each activity in the medical stream is associated with a particular socioeconomic result: medical services and other resources are used, the patient's level of social, personal, or employment functioning is altered, and so on. The task of a socioeconomic evaluation is to delineate and quantify where possible this latter stream of events.

Through socioeconomic evaluations, it is possible to make better informed decisions regarding the use, distribution, and financing of health care services and technologies. Although socioeconomic evaluations are not a panacea for rising health care costs, they provide information which health care decision-makers can use to help optimize their resource allocation decisions.

Socioeconomic evaluations in health care are used to help decision-makers make informed resource allocation decisions about health care technologies such as medications.

Types of Socioeconomic Evaluation

There are several types of evaluation to estimate the socioeconomic effects of medical technologies. They are distinguished primarily by the kind of cost and consequence measured and the methods used to measure them. Three types of study assess both the costs and consequences of medical interventions: cost-benefit, cost-effectiveness, and cost-utility analysis.

In *cost-benefit analysis* (CBA), the costs and the consequences of a technology are expressed in monetary terms. This often entails placing a monetary value on health outcomes. Because all consequences are valued in the same metric, CBAs allow comparisons of disparate types of interventions with widely divergent outcomes. For example, it would be theoretically possible to compare the construction of a hospital with the construction of a dam. One drawback of CBA is, however, that not all consequences are easily estimated in monetary terms, and placing monetary values on changes in the quality of human lives can be particularly problematic. Furthermore, consequences that are not easily expressed in monetary terms may be ignored in a CBA, thus potentially misstating the true consequences of an intervention.

A cost-benefit analysis compares two or more technologies and expresses both inputs and outcomes in monetary terms.

Cost-effectiveness analysis (CEA) was developed to address this limitation of CBA. It has been used extensively in medical care. In CEA, input costs are measured in monetary terms but health outcomes or consequences are measured in their natural units such as number of lives saved, years of life saved, cases diagnosed, or cases prevented. The strength of CEA lies in that no dollar value is placed on human life or health outcomes. It is obvious that economic costs are not a valid representation of the entire effects of a treatment and that decisions should not be based solely on considerations of cost, unless all other consequences are the same between the alternatives being compared.

Cost-effectiveness analysis compares two or more technologies, measuring the inputs in monetary terms and the outcomes in natural units such as years of life saved.

Although CEA allows researchers to examine the cost per unit of health outcome, only interventions whose outcomes are measured in equivalent units can be compared. For example, in a CEA, it is assumed that all years of life are equivalent: adding 10 years to one person's life has the same value as adding 1 year of life for ten people. Where this assumption manifestly cannot be made, the CEA approach cannot be used: a year in the life of a debilitated cancer victim is, for example, unlikely to be considered as equivalent to a year in the life of a patient with simple high blood pressure.

Cost-utility analysis (CUA) addresses this limitation of CEA by measuring the "utility" or value of years of life rather than just enumerating them. Outcomes are measured in terms of their quality or utility, which is an explicit nonmonetary valuation of various aspects of outcome. One drawback of this method is that the field of utility analysis is relatively young and the methodology is still developing. Unlike the use of CEA, which can examine a number of intermediate health outcomes such as cases found or cases prevented, there is only one outcome measure in CUA: quality-adjusted life years (QALYs).

Cost-utility analysis compares two or more interventions. Like CBA and CEA, inputs are measured in monetary terms, but outcomes are measured in terms of their quality or utility.

Other types of socioeconomic evaluation are also discussed in Part I. These include *cost-minimization analysis* (CMA), *cost-of-illness (COI) studies,* and *quality of life (QOL) assessments.* CMAs concentrate on the health care costs associated with interventions and are generally useful only when efficacy is similar or identical for each of the interventions being compared. This is rarely the case. COI studies estimate the total economic impact of a disease or a condition as opposed to the costs of an intervention for the disease. QOL studies measure the impact of conditions or treatments on the total personal and social well-being of patients.

These various types of socioeconomic evaluation attempt to measure the social and economic effect of diseases or their treatments. They step beyond an assessment of the clinical efficacy of a treatment (such as a medication) and attempt to understand the effects of treatments in a much broader sense. The specific formulation used in a study depends on the problem to be analyzed, the data that are available, and the valuation methods that will be used. One type of socioeconomic evaluation is not inherently better or worse than another. However, in any particular case, one method is likely to be more appropriate than another according to the type of question asked and the type of data which are available.

> The choice of which type of socioeconomic evaluation to perform is guided by a number of factors: the objectives of the study, the available interventions, the clinical problem, the data that are available, and the acceptability of various ways in which outcomes can be valued (for example, monetarily, in natural units, or in terms of patient preferences).

The Research Question

A socioeconomic evaluation begins with a clinically based hypothesis and a research question which states the objective of the study. The research question outlines the *alternatives* that will be examined, the *perspective* taken, and the *pathway of clinical management* that will be considered.

Asking the Right Question. It is not normally the *analyst* who poses the initial research question. Rather it is posed by a client decision-maker, sometimes a clinical decision-maker, more often a manager or producer. Occasionally the analyst may also be a decision-maker – in which case his role as one should be kept distinct from his role as the other. The early stage of research design in which the guiding research question is asked is a crucial stage and requires much consultation between analysts and "clients". It often turns out that the question initially in the minds of decision-makers was not the question that they *really* needed help with, or that the initial question was too *imprecise* to form the basis of a well-focussed study, or that the original research question soon becomes *superseded* by another more pressing one. Early joint brainstorming between analysts and clients is an important phase therefore in clarifying the question and making sure that the one finally settled on is answerable in sufficient detail to be useful, and embodies the concerns and objectives that are really those of the client. Even when there is no clearly definable client, it is important for analysts to conduct an imaginary dialogue with imagined clients in order to clarify the issues to be addressed. Failure to address the right question and failure to address any specific question clearly enough have proved potent sources for the failure of many studies to have impact on practice. Moreover, when there is a well-defined client, he is often likely to be a major source of primary data so that an ongoing relationship between client and analysts is important for this reason as well as for helping to ensure that the project proceeds on the right (viz., relevant) track and that, when major issues of judgment or discretion require resolution, the values of clients can be properly and fully represented in the analysis.

An effective socioeconomic evaluation requires close contact between clients and analysts both at the problem-formulation stage and as the analysis proceeds.

The Socioeconomic Hypothesis. To develop relevant socioeconomic hypotheses, socioeconomic analysts must understand the clinical effects of the technology. For example, hypotheses about the likely costs and consequences of a medication are derived from clinical information on the quality, efficacy, and safety of the drug. The clinical efficacy of a drug is the basis for any socioeconomic advantages and a drug with socioeconomic advantages may lead to lower costs for outpatient care (fewer concomitant medications, fewer outpatient visits), lower inpatient costs (fewer hospitalizations, shorter lengths of stay), lower costs in the nonmedical sector of the economy (fewer days absent from work, longer productive life), and greater quality of life (improved social and emotional functioning, greater sense of well-being).

Socioeconomic analysts must understand the clinical effects of the intervention before relevant socioeconomic hypotheses can be developed.

Alternatives. Most socioeconomic evaluations compare one treatment alternative with another, even if the comparison is "no treatment." Ideally, socioeconomic evaluations should examine those alternatives that are actually available or that would be realistic options in the clinical setting. It is important that the choice of alternatives is not too narrow. For example, there may be a tendency to compare one drug against another drug when a feasible and possibly more relevant option is to compare a drug with a nondrug therapy such as surgery or behavioral/educational approaches. It is also sometimes desirable to include alternatives that seem on the face of it to be nonstarters, especially if they are supported by an important professional or politically influential group (if only to demonstrate once and for all why they are indeed nonstarters!).

The alternatives compared in a socioeconomic evaluation should represent real choices in daily clinical practice and should not ignore important competitors, even though the alternatives may represent completely different classes of intervention.

The choice of alternatives can introduce unacknowledged biases into the study: the cost-effectiveness of a particular drug depends to a large extent on the alternative analyzed. Thus, the report should justify why specific alternatives were chosen and, where appropriate, why others were not.

Perspective. Perspective refers to the viewpoint from which the study is performed; in other words, whose interests are considered in the evaluation? Perspective largely defines the types of cost and consequence that will be assessed and is also a powerful determinant of the conclusions that will be drawn from the study results. The most common perspectives are those of society, the third party payer (insurance companies or national sickness funds), and the health care provider. Studies are rarely performed from the perspective of patients alone. Generally, the societal perspective is to be preferred because it considers the general social welfare rather than only the well-being of a specific actor in the health care arena. Because studies conducted from the point of view of a specific actor will tend to examine only those costs and consequences that are relevant to their budgets, the solutions from these narrower perspectives are almost always suboptimal and may lead to wasteful decisions when examined in the context of the general social welfare. In the early phase of problem definition, the issue of perspective is the principal issue to be resolved.

> To avoid neglecting potentially important costs and consequences or the shifting of costs from one sector of society to another, decisions regarding the use and reimbursement of health care interventions should, so far as possible, be based on evaluations made from the societal perspective.

For example, a government agency in charge of decision about reimbursement for a new drug may wish to examine the impact of that drug on its own health care expenditures. Such a narrow analysis would ignore a vast array of costs and consequences that should be considered in making a judgment regarding the adoption of medications. Such costs might include nonreimbursed costs borne by the patient and his or her family, the costs covered by other third party payers, and the costs absorbed by health care providers.

Inclusion of these costs and consequences provides a much richer base of information for decision-makers, allowing them to understand the varied effects of a medication, those costs that are often hidden, and those consequences which fall outside the limited scope of the agency's perspective. Ignoring these costs and consequences can result in decisions which are not optimal for society in general. One agency's budget may benefit, but overall costs may increase. It is often erroneously assumed that the government's perspective is the same as "society's." Although this may sometimes be the case, when a specific component of the government is concerned with the impact of a new program or technology on its budget to the exclusion of all other budgets, a decidedly nonsocietal perspective has been taken and important costs (and benefits) may have been overlooked. If, after full discussion with clients, it is decided nonetheless to proceed with a study from a more restrictive viewpoint, the limitations should be stressed in the study's presentation and some indication given to the significance of any omissions.

Clinical Management Pathways. The research question also sets the parameters for the pathways of clinical management that will be assessed in the evaluation. These pathways define the clinical stream of events which form the basis for estimating the socioeconomic stream. It is at this point that the potential areas of resource use are defined. The results of the study can be altered considerably by the addition or deletion of a particular category of cost or consequence, that is, by including one pathway of clinical management rather than another. Clinical knowledge is absolutely vital at this stage of describing the pathways of clinical management because, without clinical knowledge, important inputs and outcomes may be neglected. Enough information should be provided in the research report to allow the reader to identify those significant costs and consequences that were *not* assessed and to form a view of the extent to which such omissions may compromise any results.

Fundamental Concepts of Economic Analysis

Two fundamental concepts lie at the heart of all economic analyses: opportunity cost and marginal analysis.

Opportunity Cost. The true economic cost of an intervention is the value of the benefits that would be derived from using the resources required for that intervention in their next best use. This is termed the opportunity cost. The concept of opportunity cost is the basis of the monetary valuation of medical resource use.

> The true cost of any intervention is the value of the alternative interventions which are forgone.

In a truly competitive market, prices will equal economic or opportunity costs. The medical care market, however, is not truly competitive for a number of reasons such as lack of consumer sensitivity to prices (due to health insurance coverage) and providers' control of demand for services. As a result, the prices or charges affixed to goods and services do not generally reflect their true economic value. Nonetheless, because of the difficulty of estimating the opportunity cost, most socioeconomic evaluations *faute de mieux* use prices or charges as a proxy for costs. A good analysis will, however, make some asssessment of the likely biases that such compromises between the practical and the ideal may have introduced.

Marginal Analysis. The second fundamental concept of economic analysis is marginal analysis. Generally, the basic question asssessed in socioeconomic evaluations is not *whether* to employ a particular intervention, but rather *when* to employ it, *how often,* under *what clinical conditions,* and in *what specific circumstances?* Thus, the question is, "what is the additional cost of producing more of that good or service and how much additional benefit will be derived from that level of investment?" This question deals with the *marginal* or incremental costs of an intervention and the marginal benefits that are expected.

> Marginal analysis allows the assessment of the incremental impact of investing additional resources in a technology. In this way, an estimate can be made of the effects of expanding the use of the technology to other patient groups or increasing the frequency of its use.

Although socioeconomic evaluations should ideally examine marginal costs and consequences, a major limitation is that generally only data on average costs and consequences are available. By using average rather than marginal costs and consequences, it is much more difficult to determine the optimal use of a technology. Again, any likely biases will be addressed in a good study.

Measuring Costs and Consequences

Ideally, socioeconomic evaluations should include all potentially relevant costs and consequences over all time. However, practical compromises must inevitably be made. Because of limitations in money, time, and data availability, many studies examine only those particular costs and consequences that are expected to be most salient. Researchers and clients must use judgment in simplifying a broadly stated research question into a workable study plan.

> An ideal evaluation would examine all costs and all consequences over all time compared with all relevant alternatives. Because this is impossible, a choice must be made about the most salient costs, consequences, time frame, and alternatives to examine.

Costs. There are two general categories of costs: direct costs and indirect costs. *Direct costs* include actual changes in resource use that are attributable to the medication. It is important to examine not only those direct medical costs that are associated with the drug, but to look beyond drug costs to other sectors of the health care market. *Direct nonmedical costs* include resource expenditures outside the medical care market, such as costs borne by patients in seeking care.

> Most studies do a good job of including direct medical costs; however, direct nonmedical costs such as patient transportation, out-of-pocket costs, and child care expenses are often ignored.

Direct costs are subdivided into *fixed* and *variable* costs. Variable costs vary with the volume of services rendered while fixed costs remain constant across the entire range of service volumes. By definition, variable costs such as medical supplies or medications are gained or lost depending on whether they are used and in what volumes. On the other hand, fixed costs are "fixed," that is, they cannot be "saved," at least in the short run or as a consequence of adopting an option under investigation, regardless of whether or not they are used in that option. From a policy- or decision-maker's standpoint, it is critical that costs be examined carefully to estimate which are truly variable to the program that is affected by the medical technology under study.

Less obvious but important to many comprehensive economic evaluations are *indirect costs*. Indirect costs reflect the value of changes in health status and productivity that result from the health care intervention. These costs are termed "indirect" because they are not directly expended in the production of health care services or products and are not themselves true opportunity costs of the resources used in a program. Changes in health status may be valued in monetary or nonmonetary terms. Some analysts prefer to classify these effects not as costs at all but as negative consequences (negative benefits), though the authors of this guide classify negative consequences as costs and positive consequences as benefits.

There are two main approaches to reaching the monetary value of indirect costs. First, in the *human capital approach* to measuring indirect costs, changes in productivity are measured as the average earnings of persons in the labor force that will be lost or gained as a result of using a drug. A second approach to placing a monetary value on health and life is the *willingness to pay* method which is preferred conceptually by many economists because it theoretically takes into account a broader array of costs than does the human capital approach. The willingness to pay method elicits values which individuals would spend to stay healthy. Both the human capital and willingness to pay methods can be useful in estimating the indirect costs and benefits associated with a medical intervention but both also have several ethical and analytical limitations.

> Indirect costs are important to consider in many socioeconomic evaluations because the economic impact of interventions is not limited to the immediate clinical arena.

Three major considerations dictate the type of resource change that is valued in monetary terms in a socioeconomic evaluation. These include the type of analysis to be performed, for example, cost-benefit, cost-effectiveness, or cost-utility analysis; the perspective taken in the study; and the alternatives to which the technology in question will be compared.

Consequences. The consequences of medical interventions are the clinical, psychosocial, and economic outcomes of employing that intervention. Clinical consequences include measures of death, disability, and illness. Psychosocial consequences include personal outcomes such as pain and anxiety, and social effects such as work days lost and job changes resulting from illness. Many of these outcomes were considered intangible until methodological advances such as utility measurement and quality of life assessment were made. Economic consequences are health outcomes which have been valued in monetary terms. Of course, very important economic consequences of a medical intervention are the changes in health care costs themselves: savings or additional expenditures that result from the use of particular interventions. Although the goal of socioeconomic evaluation is to assess the full range of consequences that results from the use of a medication, this is often not feasible, practical, or sometimes even necessary.

Measuring consequences is a challenging task for the researcher. Many important outcomes are not quantifiable in monetary terms, and thus cost-benefit analysis is not always possible. Clinical consequences such as morbidity and mortality may be appropriate for some research questions. However, these measures often do not capture the full range of outcomes that results from treatment, and may not describe adequately even the direct clinical consequences.

Quality of life assessment and utility analysis are means of measuring those effects that have previously been considered intangible. In quality of life studies, patients are asked to respond to a series of questions about their social, psychological, physical, and intellectual well-being in order to identify precisely what aspects of a patient's life are affected by a disease or intervention. Such studies can result in detailed accounts of the impact of interventions and can provide the basis for choosing among interventions which have very similar costs but which can have different effects on patients' personal well-being. These consequences of therapy are not assessed using typical clinical measures.

Utility analysis, on the other hand, seeks to compress these psychological effects into one summary measure in order to compare vastly divergent outcomes in terms of a common metric, usually expressed on a scale that ranges from 1 (perfect health) to 0 (death). Life-years weighted by utility values form the denominator of a cost-utility ratio, a measure that is easily grasped and which effectively summarizes the health effects in a single measure that embodies a variety of explicit trade-offs.

In general, researchers should begin a study by enumerating the full range of consequences that are based on the available clinical evidence. They should evaluate which consequences are most relevant, what weights they should receive, and which consequences are most likely to differ between the alternatives compared. They should examine consequences so as to appraise those which are appropriately measured in monetary terms, those which are to be measured in natural units, and those which can be valued using quality of life or utility measures. Finally, in reporting results, researchers should make explicit which potentially important outcomes are *not* included in the final results and what impact these omissions might have on the interpretation of results. A qualitative description of the consequences that have been excluded from the analysis is often helpful. Readers of socioeconomic studies can go through the same type of analytical process to determine whether all relevant consequences were included and adequately expressed.

> In reading a socioeconomic evaluation, it is important to assess whether the salient consequences were included in the analysis. If some important consequences are missing, readers should try to judge what impact their inclusion might have on the evaluation results.

Sensitivity Analysis

Researchers face significant challenges in accurately estimating the impact of intervention on costs and on patients' well-being. These challenges often mean that relatively gross estimates must be made and that these estimates are subject to considerable uncertainty. Assumptions must often be made regarding resource use, the costs of resources, or the health effects of an intervention. When such assumptions are made, researchers cannot be certain that their conclusions are tenable, that is, whether the conclusions are "sensitive" to changes in these assumptions. *Sensitivity analysis* is an important analytical tool which can be used to test whether the conclusions of a study change as assumptions are altered. It should always be performed whenever there is uncertainty about key variables, about how best to measure them, and about how well they have been measured.

> Socioeconomic evaluations normally include information which is subject to uncertainty. Sensitivity analysis is a vital tool which can assess how important these areas of uncertainty are and whether different assumptions or estimates would produce substantially different results.

When faced with uncertainty about the true value for some costs or consequences, researchers will generally begin by choosing a value that is a "best estimate". They will then vary that estimate, usually suggesting a high value and a low value and then repeat the calculations to see whether their results change under the high and low assumptions. If the conclusions drawn from the study do not change as these values are altered, the results of the analysis are "robust" to changes in this variable. We can accept the conclusions of the study if the sensitivity analysis encompasses the true range of possible values for that variable. If the conclusions change with sensitivity analysis, then faith in the analysis is less certain. Sensitivity analyses performed relatively early in the study may suggest to the researchers some topics on which more detailed research should be undertaken and this is a practice that should be encouraged.

Discounting

When costs or consequences do not occur within a relatively short time frame, or when costs and consequences do not occur at the same time, the results of the socioeconomic evaluation should be adjusted to reflect *positive time preference.* This means that costs and consequences incurred in the present have greater value than those which occur in the future. Basically, discounting reduces future costs and consequences to their present value by an inflation-free discount rate (usually between 3% and 5% annually).

> Discounting is another important tool that allows the analyst to incorporate future costs and consequences in socioeconomic evaluations in a way that does not overrepresent their true value.

Other Study Design Issues

Socioeconomic evaluations can be conducted by using prospective or, more commonly, retrospective data. Prospective data might be collected in conjunction with a randomized controlled trial (RCT) of a medication whereas a retrospective study uses data from existing sources, such as the clinical and economic literature or a claims data base from a third party payer.

Inclusion of economic measures and quality of life surveys within a clinical trial is relatively recent, but this practice can be expected to increase in the future. Such prospective studies can supply highly valid information because of the strength of the RCT design. However, there may be problems in generalizing the results to other patient groups. Because RCTs are expensive, they are often performed on relatively small and specialized groups of patients. Moreover they are usually performed by enthusiasts and leaders of the field in centers of excellence; therefore it is not clear that the results can be generalized to other populations or practices. On the other hand, retrospective studies often make use of large population-based data sets, or they use "best estimate" values in conjunction with analytical modeling techniques to simulate general population values. These studies suffer from a different kind of uncertainty. Because the data are seldom derived from well-controlled studies, the precision of values may suffer. Sensitivity analysis as discussed above is particularly helpful in analyzing the results and improving the "believability" of retrospective studies.

There are trade-offs in both retrospective and prospective studies. When prospective studies are based on RCTs, the information they yield is often highly accurate, but it often suffers from lack of generalizability. When retrospective studies use large data sets such as medical claims data bases, they often are generalizable to a broader population but may lack detail and accuracy.

Conclusion

Although socioeconomic evaluations attempt to measure and evaluate the costs and consequences of a medical treatment as accurately as possible, they face restrictions of having to gather data in the real world and having to draw conclusions on the basis of incomplete information. As a result, the costs measured in economic analyses are not true opportunity costs. Rather they represent either an imperfect price set in a noncompetitive marketplace or an arbitrary price set by a government commission or other proxy. Moreover, even though marginal analysis is a critical goal of an economic evaluation for optimal decision-making, average costs and consequences are usually the only costs available.

Furthermore, socioeconomic evaluations generally collect data on only the most salient costs and consequences on a few alternatives, and do so over a relatively restricted time frame. As a result, some important costs and consequences may be neglected and some important alternatives ignored. In assessing a research report it is important critically to evaluate whether significant changes might be anticipated if other costs and consequences had been incorporated and if other alternatives had been compared. The perspective of the analysis also determines the outcome of a study to a large extent. Studies conducted from the perspective of society take into account costs and consequences regardless of to whom they accrue. Therefore, they are least likely to result in a shifting of costs from one segment of society to another.

Socioeconomic evaluations are important tools for decision-makers in the health care field. Health care decision-makers face increasingly difficult choices between competing alternatives, such as choices between medications with apparently equivalent efficacy. If these choices are based simply on a comparison of the monetary costs per dose of the drugs, other important costs and consequences may be disregarded: these include costs such as those associated with the utilization of medical resources to treat significant adverse reactions, or consequences such as differences in quality of life. Socioeconomic evaluations can provide balanced and impartial appraisals of the relative costs and efficacy of interventions and are increasingly essential tools for decision-making.

Part I

Guidelines for the Evaluator

1 Introduction to Socioeconomic Evaluations

1.1 Introduction

As health care costs have skyrocketed during the past two decades, governments and private industry have made repeated attempts to curtail this escalation through regulation and planning efforts with limited success. One path to controlling health care costs is to invest only in those technologies which can provide benefits at least as large as their costs.

Socioeconomic evaluations[1] help one draw conclusions about the costs and benefits of medical services such as medications. These techniques make it possible to compare medical services and to discern which ones will result in the greatest benefit for the costs. This book describes these socioeconomic evaluation methods and the research processes involved.

Socioeconomic evaluations:

Research methods which assess the costs and/or consequences of medical technologies in order to compare alternatives.

This text focusses on the evaluation of medications, although the principles and guidelines presented apply to other health care technologies as well. The choice of medications as an example is particularly apt because the pharmaceutical industry is experiencing intense market pressure for cost containment. Pharmaceutical firms are increasingly performing socioeconomic evaluations on their products and the results of evaluations are being used by health policymakers to make decisions about the relative clinical and socioeconomic value of medications.

1.2 Brief History of Socioeconomic Evaluations

The common sense principles of socioeconomic evaluations have been promoted for centuries, and application of these principles to health care dates back at least 300 years. In the middle of the seventeenth century, Richard Petty, a prominent

[1] The most commonly performed socioeconomic evaluations are cost-benefit and cost-effectiveness analysis, which are described in detail in Chap. 3.

English physician, concluded that the value of human lives saved as a result of greater social investment in health care far exceeded the cost.

Use of formal socioeconomic evaluations was not widespread until the twentieth century. Before the 1960s, the techniques of socioeconomic evaluation were used by US Army Corps of Engineers, which developed most of the water projects in the United States. In the 1960s, the US Department of Defense adopted a program-budgeting system that employed cost-benefit analysis to evaluate alternative defense projects. The perception that these evaluations assisted in rational defense planning, combined with a growing federal budget, led President Johnson in 1965 to require the implementation of similar evaluation systems throughout the federal bureaucracy. The principles of socioeconomic evaluation were applied to other public works projects such as transportation, urban renewal, health, education, and income maintenance. Prominent examples of health care socioeconomic evaluations during this period were the studies of efforts to control kidney disease, maternal and child health care programs, health services for the poor, and nursing personnel programs.

The health program of the US Office of Technology Assessment (OTA) produced the most comprehensive study of socioeconomic evaluations in health care in 1980 and examined the cost-effectiveness of several specific medical technologies. One such study, a cost-effectiveness analysis of pneumococcal vaccine, played a central role in legislation, permitting Medicare to reimburse health care providers for pneumococcal vaccinations.

Interest in socioeconomic evaluations has grown rapidly among health policy decisions-makers, health care administrators, and medical practitioners not only in the United States but also internationally. In general, the interest stems from concern about the mounting costs of health services, increased governmental spending, and the perception that the allocation of health care resources must be rationalized. Groups as disparate as providers and third-party payers have expressed a desire for cost-effectiveness information to aid them in promoting greater efficiency in the provision of health care services.

Growth of interest in health care socioeconomic evaluations is a phenomenon of the 1970s and the 1980s. There has been a continued acceleration in the number of articles devoted to socioeconomic evaluations and in the types of medical interventions which have been assessed. Pharmaceutical manufacturers are increasingly interested in evaluations of their products. The US Health Care Financing Administration may soon require socioeconomic evaluations as part of the approval process for reimbursing the costs of some medications.

Considerable methodological advances have been made in the techniques of socioeconomic evaluation and guidelines have been provided by the OTA regarding ideal standards. Nonetheless, there is still considerable disparity in the quality of studies and there appear to be some barriers to the application of the results of socioeconomic evaluations. This may be attributed to several problems. First, there is a wide variety of socioeconomic evaluation techniques which can be applied to a particular problem, and each evaluation can be conducted in a number of ways. Second, researchers labor under significant limitations regarding data availability and the resources needed to conduct studies. This means that research results are less than perfect and the results of an evaluation do not always point to straightforward solutions to complex problems. Researchers conducting socioeconomic evaluations must make important compromises and choices. In turn, readers and users of socioeconomic evaluations must remain aware of these compromises and choices and should ideally be actively involved in the judgements that are made when such compromises are unavoidable.

1.3 Compromises and Choices in Socioeconomic Evaluation

Two major themes recur throughout this book: One deals with the inevitable need for compromise in translating the ideal research plan into a practicable study. The other theme deals with the importance of careful choices in developing the research design and in conducting socioeconomic evaluations. While at first these themes seem to conflict, they are both of critical importance in conducting evaluations that are both timely and successful.

The first theme, the need for compromise, is illustrated throughout this book in examples where the ideal is juxtaposed with the practical, and the exemplary is contrasted with the expedient. Because it is impossible for every study to adhere perfectly to the most pristine standards of research design, data collection, analysis, and interpretation, compromises must inevitably be made in what is measured and how it is measured. The guidelines or standards presented here can be used in the critical assessment of reported research studies and to determine when compromises are unavoidable, how they may best be made and, at the end of the day, whether the compromises were actually appropriately executed.

Socioeconomic evaluations seek to assess the impact that medications have on individuals and on society. This impact pertains not only to the biomedical effect of medications (which is the focus of clinical studies), but also to the effects of medications on individuals' well-being, their economic productivity, and their ability to perform their normal social roles. Socioeconomic evaluations also describe how the use of a medication may shift resources from one sector of the economy to another, how it may increase or decrease hospitalization, and how it may affect the use of other treatment services, immediately and in the future.

Ideally, a socioeconomic evaluation should study all the resources required to provide a treatment, all the benefits that a person receives, all the medical side effects that patients experience, all the effects on patients' personal lives and their social interactions, and all the influences on the economy in general. Any study could thus be almost limitless in its scope, and its cost could be staggering. Researchers must decide which are the most important inputs and outcomes relevant to the specific technology being evaluated, which data are most vital to collect, and what is the most feasible way of obtaining the data. Choices must be made at each stage of the evaluation process. It is in this translation from the ideal to the pragmatic that compromises must be made.

Some compromises represent acceptable options and, given the appropriate precautions, these studies can yield tenable conclusions. In other cases, the compromises are unreasonable and meaningful conclusions cannot at all be drawn from the study. In still other cases, there is too little information in the report to enable the reader critically to assess whether the compromises made in the study were appropriate. It is critical that the compromises are stated explicitly in the study report and, if there are direct clients for its results, that their perspective be crusidered in the process of making any necessary compromises on what is ideal.

This book will describe the standards or principles of socioeconomic evaluation. Common compromises will be explained. Generally accepted compromises will be distinguished from those which stray too far from the standards to allow the results of the study to be accepted with confidence. While specific techniques of data acquisition and analysis will change as the field develops, these standards are fundamental. It is hoped that readers will be able to assess a report of an evaluation critically, discern whether a study adhered to the essential guidelines that are expected of any evaluation, judge the value of the results, and assess whether the study addressed the particular policy concerns of interest.

The second theme of this book, choice, is more specific to socioeconomic evaluations. In acknowledging the need for compromises, researchers must choose the types of costs and benefits which should be examined and how those costs and benefits will be measured and assigned values. There are numerous determinants of how these choices are made. First, researchers make basic choices when they determine the type of study to be used to perform the socioeconomic evaluation. Should it be a cost-benefit or cost-effectiveness analysis? Should the effect of this medication be assessed with a quality of life study? Is it adequate to perform a cost-minimization analysis? Depending on the type of study chosen, costs and benefits are measured in certain ways and, in some studies, one or the other may not be measured at all.

When researchers set the framework for an evaluation they necessarily make further choices which narrow the scope of their activity and reduce it to a manageable task. They must pose a specific research question which limits the types of cost and outcome which they will measure. They must choose a perspective from which the study will be performed, they must choose specific alternatives to which the medication will be compared, and they must describe the range of inputs and outputs which will fall within the scope of the study. As with compromises, researchers' judgments on all these matters are best made considering the perspective of potential clients.

In choosing the study design, researchers further define the costs and benefits that will be included and how they will be measured. Within a prospective study design, for which data are collected after the study begins, researchers will have greater latitude in designating which costs and benefits to include. Retrospective studies, by contrast, are limited in the type of variables that can be examined and measured because the rely upon previously collected data.

These two themes, that compromises are necessary and that choices must be made among alternative evaluation approaches, are linked by the restrictions placed on researchers when they translate their ideas for a study to its practical performance. These restrictions include the availability of research funds, time, and data. Researchers must take advantage of opportunities such as ongoing clinical trials within which to collect socioeconomic data or the availability of a large medical claims data base. Often, however, such opportunities do not exist and alternatives must be sought. All of these choices mold the research study into a workable project, but at the same time these choices present pitfalls. The standards described should assist in identifying and avoiding these pitfalls. The basic question is: Were the appropriate choices made for the goals the researchers set out to accomplish? A second and equally critical question is: Were the researcher's goals appropriate: Did they ask the most critical questions and did they address the most important issues in examining a particular intervention?

1.4 Why Socioeconomic Evaluations Are Performed

Medications and medical devices are routinely evaluated for their clinical efficacy and safety. Traditionally, if a treatment did what it purported to do, then it was apparently worthy of use. However, the medical care marketplace and its political, social, demographic, and economic environments in Western countries have changed considerably in the past 20 years.

There are five major changes:

1. An aging population
2. An increase in the number and types of health care professionals
3. Continued development of medical technologies (medications, devices, and procedures)
4. Increasing public demands for improved quality of medical care
5. Pressures in all countries to constrain the growth of expenditures for medical care.

These first four changes mean that the demand for health care will continue to increase. They are countered by the fifth change. One way to reduce health care expenditures is to limit access to medical care services. Another is to make sure that the money that society spends for health care is spent wisely. This means that medical services and products such as medications are being analyzed more closely.

1.5 Organization of the Text

Part I provides a discussion of the details of the evaluation process. The standards of socioeconomic evaluation are presented and the common compromises are reviewed.

In Chapter 2, several important concepts are discussed which underlie socioeconomic evaluation: costs, consequences, and the time dimension. Chapter 3 describes the major study types or forms of socioeconomic evaluation and presents examples of each study type. Chapter 4 provides an understanding of the basic framework of socioeconomic evaluations: the formulation of the research question, the perspective, the alternatives compared, and the production relationship. Chapter 5 details types of costs and their valuation, with a focus on commonly encountered problems. Chapter 6 describes the identification of the health and economic consequences of therapy. Methods of adjusting costs and consequences for time and uncertainty are described in Chapter 7. Study design issues are discussed in Chapter 8. Chapter 9 is a summary, with a checklist that can be used by readers to assess socioeconomic evaluations and two examples of such assessments. Examples of specific studies are used throughout the text.

Part II details the technical aspects of several important methods used in socioeconomic evaluations. Chapters 10 through 14 provide further clarification of key concepts and indepth coverage of topics such as utility analysis, quality of life, decision analysis, and statistical methods.

2 Concepts in Socioeconomic Evaluation

2.1 Introduction

The introduction and use of a medication has several potential effects, which are illustrated in Fig. 2.1. The main purpose of a health care intervention such as a medication (box A) is usually to create positive changes in health status (box B). Such changes can be measured as reductions in an undesired health state (morbidity and mortality) or increases in a desired one (quality of life).

Health status changes have three potential economic consequences. First, there is the inherent value of health (box C), which may be measured in terms of patients' preferences for being in healthier states. These preferences can be expressed in either economic or noneconomic terms. Second, changes in health status can be reflected in productivity changes (box D) which are also usually measured in economic terms. Healthy people work more and do so more productively. Third, changes in health status often result in a change in the utilization of

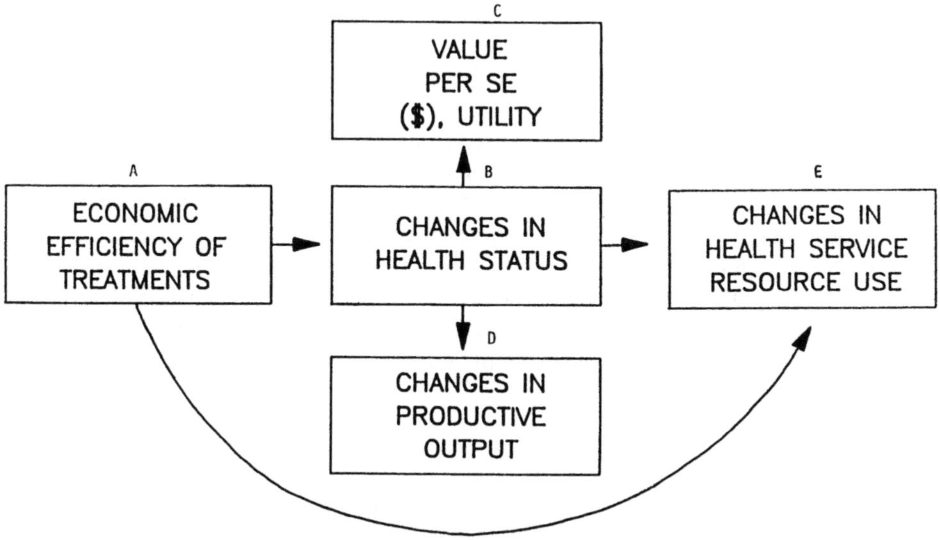

Fig. 2.1. Measuring economic efficiency in health care. (Adapted from Fig. 4.2 in Drummond 1980)

health care resources (box E); healthy people may consume fewer medical services[1].

The economic effect of a medication may be traced along another pathway. The medication can have direct effects on the distribution and use of health care resources irrespective of its clinical value. The use of a new technology may diminish the use of competing or substitute technologies or it may increase the use of complementary technologies (pathway A to E). All of the consequences occur over time, sometimes over a lifetime. Figure 2.1 does not depict the time dimension.

2.2 Generating Socioeconomic Hypotheses

A vital component of the socioeconomic evaluation of medications is the generation of hypotheses at the beginning of the analysis. The clinical consequences of a medication are the basis of hypotheses regarding its socioeconomic effects; therefore, this step requires substantial involvement of clinical experts who are knowledgeable in the use and effects of the medication.

One way to conceptualize this hypothesis generation process is through a framework called QESUNC[2] (Wernli and Sproll 1988). First of all, a drug must be of sufficient quality (Q), efficacy (E), and safety (S) to warrant approval for clinical use. This information is the basis of preclinical and clinical trials of the medication. In order to distinguish itself relative to other medications, it should perform comparably or, in some way, better than other drugs currently available. For example, the new drug may cause fewer side effects, it may have a longer half-life (thus requiring less frequent dosing), or it may be active against a broader range of pathogens or symptoms than the currently available medication. A drug's quality, efficacy, and safety are then the basis of conclusions regarding the drug's therapeutic usefulness (U) and the clinical need (N) for the drug. This information is derived from pharmacological and epidemiological information as well as the drug's clinical trials. These steps are the starting point for the socioeconomic evaluation process.

Meaningful hypotheses that are designed to test the costs and benefits (C) of a medication are derived from clinical information on the quality, efficacy, and safety of the drug. Differences in safety and efficacy can be reflected in socioeconomic differences between the two drugs. A drug with socioeconomic advantages may lead to lower costs for outpatient care (fewer concomitant medications, fewer outpatient visits), lower inpatient costs (fewer hospitalizations, shorter lengths of stay), lower costs in the nonmedical sector of the economy (fewer days absent from work, longer productive life), and greater quality of life

---

[1] This may not hold true under two conditions. Healthy people may not consume fewer medical resources than sick people if access to medical services for both groups is unequal. Furthermore, depending on the life span of the healthy and the ill individuals, healthy people living a long life may consume more medical resources than sick individuals who die at a younger age.
[2] This concept is attributed to Guenther Lewandowski, former vice president Bundesgesundheitsamt, FRG.

(improved social and emotional functioning, greater sense of well-being). In sum, socioeconomic analysts must first understand the clinical effects of the medication in order to develop relevant socioeconomic hypotheses.

2.3 Socioeconomic Concepts

Several basis concepts are central to understanding and performing socioeconomic analysis. These concepts stem from social science disciplines, primarily sociology, psychology, and economics as well as operations research and clinical decision analysis.

2.3.1 Costs

Costs are the inputs required to produce a particular outcome. In the socioeconomic evaluation of medications, costs are the resources expended to obtain a desired state of health.

Costs:

The economic inputs required to achieve a certain output.

For example, when a patient with an elevated temperature visits a physician, certain diagnostic laboratory and X-ray examinations may be undertaken to help define the problem and a medication might be prescribed to fight an infection. During this process, medical resources are expended and might include:

1. The physician's time
2. Activities of the physician's ancillary staff
3. Use of medical office space
4. Laboratory and X-ray facilities, personnel, and supplies
5. Acquisition costs of the medication
6. Storage costs of the medication
7. The pharmacist's time
8. Patient's time away from work or family
9. Cost of patient transportation to the office.

From this list, it is apparent that the costs of the antibiotic (5) are likely to be a small portion of the costs of this medical episode. If the analyst attempted to calculate *all* the costs involved in even this simple episode of outpatient care, the task would be monumental. The problem is considerably more complex when the focus is on a long hospitalization or a chronic disease that requires resource expenditures over a lifetime. As will be seen in later chapters, many compromises must be made in socioeconomic evaluations in order to expedite the research process. Rather than attempting to measure all costs, researchers often approximate some forms of costs and disregard others that are likely to be inconsequential. In the identification and approximate measurement of costs, opportunity cost is a critical concept.

Opportunity Costs. Whenever resources are devoted to the production or use of a new technology, those resources cannot be invested in other sectors of the health care economy or the economy in general. Thus, the potential benefits which may be derived from the use of limited resources in some other way are forgone. This is termed the *opportunity cost.* Opportunity costs are taken into account in socioeconomic evaluations because decisions must be made between alternative uses for scarce resources.

Opportunity Cost:

The true cost of any resource is the value of the alternative outputs that are forgone; those resources expended on a project which are not available for investment in other projects.

Scarcity of resources is at the foundation of all economic assessments, including those of medical technologies. The true economic cost of a medication is the value of the resources invested in that new medication which are no longer available for use in other activities. In a completely competitive market, the price of any product will equal its (marginal) opportunity cost; thus, the analysis of costs is greatly simplified. But when the market diverges from the ideal of competition, prices or charges no longer represent the true costs of that product. This divergence results in a difference between the economic costs and the financial (or accounting) costs of a product. The price of a technology is then only a gross proxy – and perhaps a poor one – of its opportunity cost.

In the medical care market, this divergence of market price and true cost is attributable to two distorting factors: Less lucrative products and services are *cross-subsidized* by the earnings on more profitable ones; *Cost-shifting* occurs to some patients and their third party payers from those who cannot pay all or part of their medical care bills.

Despite the obvious superiority of using opportunity costs, they are rarely used because of the difficulties in their estimation. Most socioeconomic evaluations generally employ average prices (or charges) of goods and services to represent the costs of these items, and they use wage rates to represent the opportunity cost of personnel time and effort.

Transfer Payments. Before leaving the topic of costs, the distinction between transfer payments and economic costs should be made. In a socioeconomic evaluation, only real economic costs should be included in the analysis. Real *economic costs* include only those resources that are used or lost as a result of the illness or treatment. *Transfers* include expenditures such as welfare payments, disability payments, and taxes. These do not represent the use of resources but are only a redistribution of purchasing power.

Transfer Payments:

Expenditures which are a redistribution of purchasing power rather than resources actually used or lost in the production of a service or product.

The only costs that should be included are those which reflect actual productive use of resources, not simply money that is transferred from one sector of the economy to another. Nonetheless, transfer payments may be of great interest to particular parties involved. For example, the government of a country may be interested in the budgetary consequences of changes in disability payments that may result from certain therapies. Depending on the audience for the study, transfer payments may be included in the analysis; however, they should be reported separately from the real costs and benefits.

2.3.2 Consequences

In socioeconomic evaluations, *consequences* are the results of using a medical technology, that is, the outcomes of using particular resources. The years of life saved as a result of the medication, the side effects associated with its use, and the medical care services used or saved because of the medication are all consequences. Generally, consequences are referred to as "benefits"; however, because some consequences may be negative, the term "benefits" will not be used here.

Consequences:

The outcomes that result from using a product or a service.

Many consequences are not easily measured in monetary terms, for example, years of life that are saved, the discomfort or relief caused by a medication, and the subjective feelings that patients have during or after treatment. Two major concepts are used in socioeconomic evaluations to measure these noneconomic consequences: length of life and quality of life.

Length of Life. When two treatments are compared, it may be possible to measure the consequences of using the treatment as the effect on the length of patients' lives. This is termed *life-years saved* or *years of life saved* (YOLS). Rather than attempting to quantify this consequence in monetary terms, it is possible to compare treatments that have similar outcomes using these natural units. One problem with using life-years saved as a measure of consequences is that it amounts to assuming that the quality or "importance" of each year of life across all the patients is identical. When this is not a tenable assumption, then attempts must be made to measure the difference in the *quality* of those life years.

The concepts of life years saved and quality of life are combined in *quality-adjusted life years* (QALYs). QALY – analysts are able more accurately to describe the impact of a medication on a patient's longevity and on the value of the additional life-years. QALYs and the measurement of patient preferences in the form of utilities are discussed in Chapters 3, 6, and 12.

Quality of Life. This is defined as people's abilities and perceptions that affect their performance of expected duties, their views of life, and their satisfaction and happiness. Quality of life has been conceptualized as falling into several major dimensions. One typology that has been frequently used in research studies divides quality of life into social, physical, emotional, and intellectual functioning. A global measure of general well-being is also included (Levine and Croog 1984).

All of these individual components of quality of life are related to one another. For example, a person with impaired emotional functioning such as depression may have reduced intellectual functioning, physical symptoms, and a poor sense of general well-being. By keeping these concepts separate, it is possible to identify the specific aspects of a person's life that are most affected by an illness or a medical intervention.

2.3.3 Marginal Analysis

Another important foundation of socioeconomic evaluation is the concept of *marginal analysis.* In any resource allocation decision, the goal is to maximize benefit given the scare resources available to invest in a technology or program. In order to make this decision, it is necessary to examine the marginal effects of additional increases in resource expenditure.

Marginal Analysis:

An analytical technique which examines the relationship between incremental changes in investment in a product and incremental changes in outputs.

Figure 2.2 compares the marginal benefit received from a medication to its costs. Consider the example of a new cholesterol-lowering medication which is

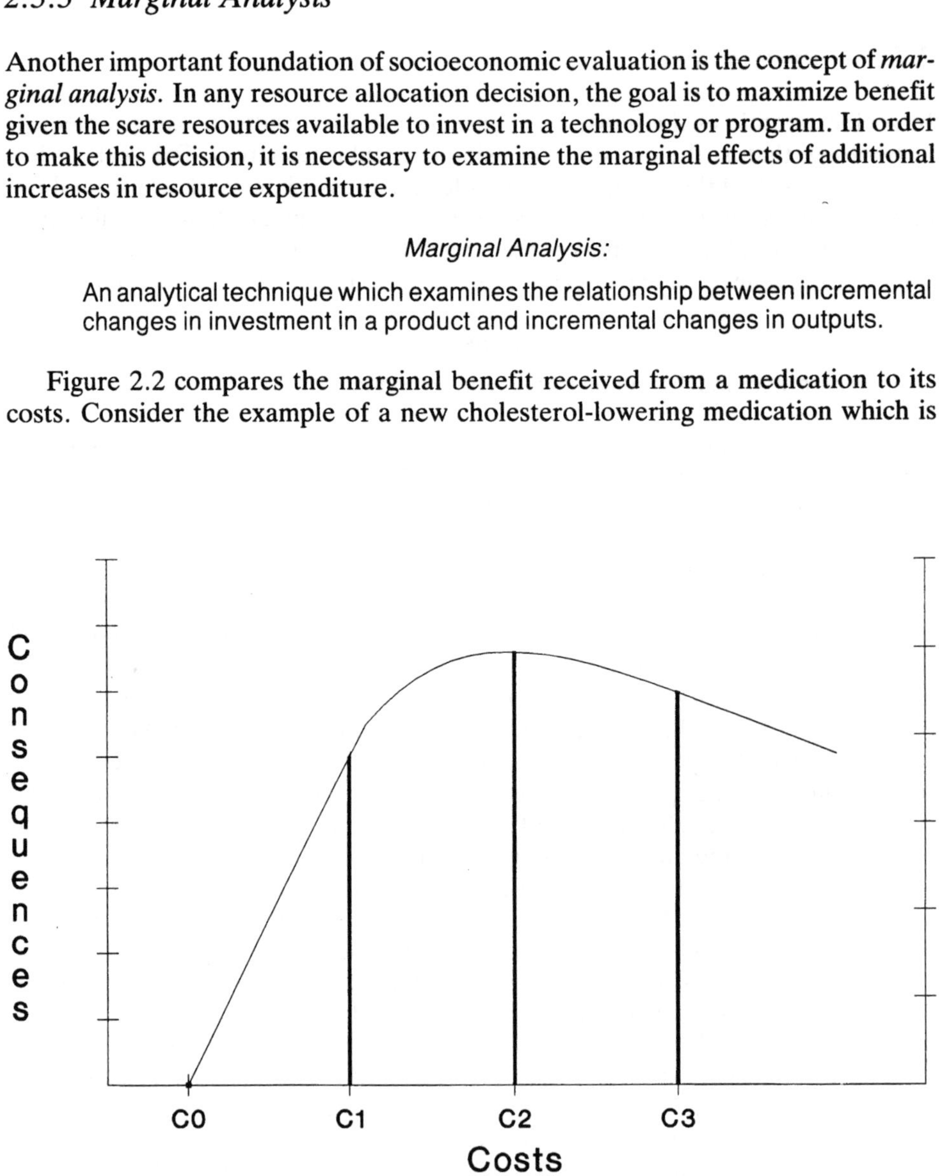

Fig. 2.2. Marginal analysis

introduced into the health care market. Assume that consequences are measured as the positive effects of lowered death and illness rates as well as the negative effects of adverse reactions to the drug. Over the first range of investment (between C0 and C1), there is a dramatic rise in benefits. In this stage, the drug may be used only for those patients with the highest serum cholesterol levels, and their levels are considerably reduced, which results in lower morbidity and mortality as a consequence of stroke and heart disease. Whatever side effects are produced by the drug are greatly outweighed by the increased life expectancy. As more economic resources are invested in the drug (C1 to C2), it is used for patients with lower cholesterol levels. There is still a marginal increase in benefits; however, the rise is not nearly so sharp as before. When even more resources are invested (C2 to C3), the drug may be used for patients with only slightly increased levels, and the additional benefits of reduced mortality and morbidity are offset by the negative consequences of side effects. It is possible to imagine a stage in which the negative effects are sufficient to outweigh positive effects altogether, with the curve actually dropping below the horizontal axis (not shown in Fig. 2.2).

In comparing the marginal worth of medications, it is possible to see how much benefit can be derived from incremental changes in investment. For example, consider two vaccines A and B. Table 2.1 depicts the total and marginal investment in each vaccine along with the benefits received from various levels of investment.

Table 2.1. Total and marginal costs of vaccines

	Vaccine A		Vaccine B	
Total cost	$100 000		$100 000	
Cases prevented		10		12
Marginal cost (first investment)	$ 50 000		$ 50 000	
Cases prevented		8		6
Marginal cost (second investment)	$ 50 000		$ 50 000	
Cases prevented		2		6

The total level of investment in each is $100 000. Vaccine A results in 10 cases prevented, while vaccine B results in 12 cases prevented. Based on these facts, we would tend to invest only in vaccine B; however, a marginal analysis leads to a vastly different conclusion. While it is true that, other things being equal, vaccine B is more efficient, a combination of some use of A and some use of B might be still more efficient.

For the first $50 000 invested in vaccine A, eight cases are prevented. When our investment increases to $100 000, a total of ten cases are prevented. The marginal benefit for an additional $50 000 was only two cases. On the other hand, the first $50 000 invested in vaccine B results in six cases being prevented. If we had only $100 000 to spend, a rational decision based on this marginal analysis would lead us to invest $50 000 in vaccine A to prevent 8 cases, and invest the remaining $50 000 in vaccine B to prevent 6 more cases, resulting in 14 cases prevented for $100 000.

By using marginal analysis in socioeconomic evaluations we do not ask "is the technology worthwhile?" Rather we ask,
"To what extent should the technology be employed?"
"When should this medication be used?"
"For what clinical condition or what severity of illness?"
"In what dosages?"
"How long should it be continued?" (Drummond et al. 1988)

A problem that arises in economic analysis is that data concerning the marginal benefits and costs of technologies are rarely available. More likely, information is available regarding the *average* benefits and *average* costs of a technology. Unfortunately, average costs may be a poor proxy for marginal costs.

Marginal Costs Versus Average Costs:

In a study of the costs of screening for occult blood in stool, which might indicate the presence of colorectal cancer, it was concluded that the *average cost* per year of life saved was $2451. Costs were then computed for multiple screening tests performed on the same person. The *marginal cost* per year of life saved when one screening test was performed was only $294. However, as subsequent tests were performed on the same individuals, cost-effectiveness declined. The marginal cost per year of life saved with the fifth test was over $1 million, while the marginal cost for the sixth test was nearly $12 million. (Neuhauser and Lewicki 1975)

There are two main reasons why marginal costs are preferable to average costs in a socioeconomic evaluation.

1. Marginal costs are more informative in providing guidelines for the efficient use of alternative technologies.
2. Marginal costs may vary a great deal with the level of utilization, and so the use of average costs can be very misleading. The same is also true when capital costs are large.

2.4 Discounting and the Dimension of Time

Fundamental to any socioeconomic evaluation is a consideration of the impact of the passage of time on the accounting of costs and consequences. Although this topic will be discussed in greater technical detail in Chap. 7, a basic understanding of the concept is necessary for understanding the next chapters. Essentially, costs or consequences that occur in the future have less value than costs and consequences that occur now. It would be preferable to receive $100 now as opposed to $100 in 10 years because that money could be invested now and interest could be earned on it. In order to take into account the effect of time, analysts *discount* future costs and consequences to their present value. A typical discount rate is 5%. This means that $100 next year will have a discounted value of $95.24 now.

2.5 Conclusion

This chapter has examined several concepts that are basic to socioeconomic evaluations. These concepts include costs, opportunity costs, consequences, marginal analysis, and discounting. Although analysts attempt to measure and evaluate the costs and consequences of a medical treatment as accurately as possible, they face restrictions of having to gather data in the real world and having to draw conclusions on the basis of incomplete information. As a result, the costs measured in most economic analyses do not measure true opportunity costs; rather, they represent the price in the marketplace.

The consequences of socioeconomic evaluations may be valued in monetary terms or in natural units. A study might examine the years of life that are saved as a result of using a medication. Alternatively, if there are differences in the quality of those life-years, then quality of life should be measured; however, in most instances this will require the collection of primary data, a luxury that cannot always be afforded. Finally, even though marginal analysis is the goal of an economic evaluation, average costs and average consequences are usually examined. It is important to be aware that relying on average costs and consequences can seriously distort an analysis and may lead to suboptimal decision-making.

3 Types of Socioeconomic Evaluation

3.1 Introduction

Socioeconomic evaluations are not a replacement for clinical research that assesses the efficacy of medications; rather, they are an adjunct to clinical or biomedical research. Socioeconomic evaluation techniques bring useful additional information to guide coverage policy, reimbursement, and clinical decisions. While biomedical research is aimed at providing evidence for the clinical efficacy of medications, socioeconomic evaluations examine the effects of drugs on a much broader range of factors including:

1. the use and cost of medical resources
2. the use and cost of resources outside the medical care market
3. the value of wages lost as a result of illness or disability
4. the patients' social, emotional and physical well-being.

3.2 Types of Socioeconomic Evaluation

Socioeconomic evaluations of medications can be thought of as methods for assessing the value of a drug. At the top of Fig. 3.1 is the general equation representing socioeconomic evaluations. The value of a drug (V_d) is equal to the sum of all costs (C) subtracted from all consequences (B,) discounted over time (t)[1] at a particular discount rate (n).

Because it is often either impossible or impractical to examine all costs and all consequences over all time, it is necessary to go through a simplification step. This occurs in the second part of Fig. 3.1. In this step, we outline those *relevant* costs and consequences that occur during a relevant period within the context of a specific study formulation. (These formulations are described later in this chapter). In order to reduce the problem to one that can be investigated given the analytical tools available, a further simplification step occurs. This is illustrated at the bottom of Fig. 3.1, where the analyst takes stock of the data and the study populations that are available and the level of uncertainty in the field. The result

[1] Discounting is achieved through the denominator of the equation, $(1 + n)^t$. Essentially, discounting means that future costs and benefits are adjusted to their present value. Costs and benefits that occur in the future have less value in present dollars. This is explained in greater detail in Chap. 7, "Adjusting Costs and Consequences."

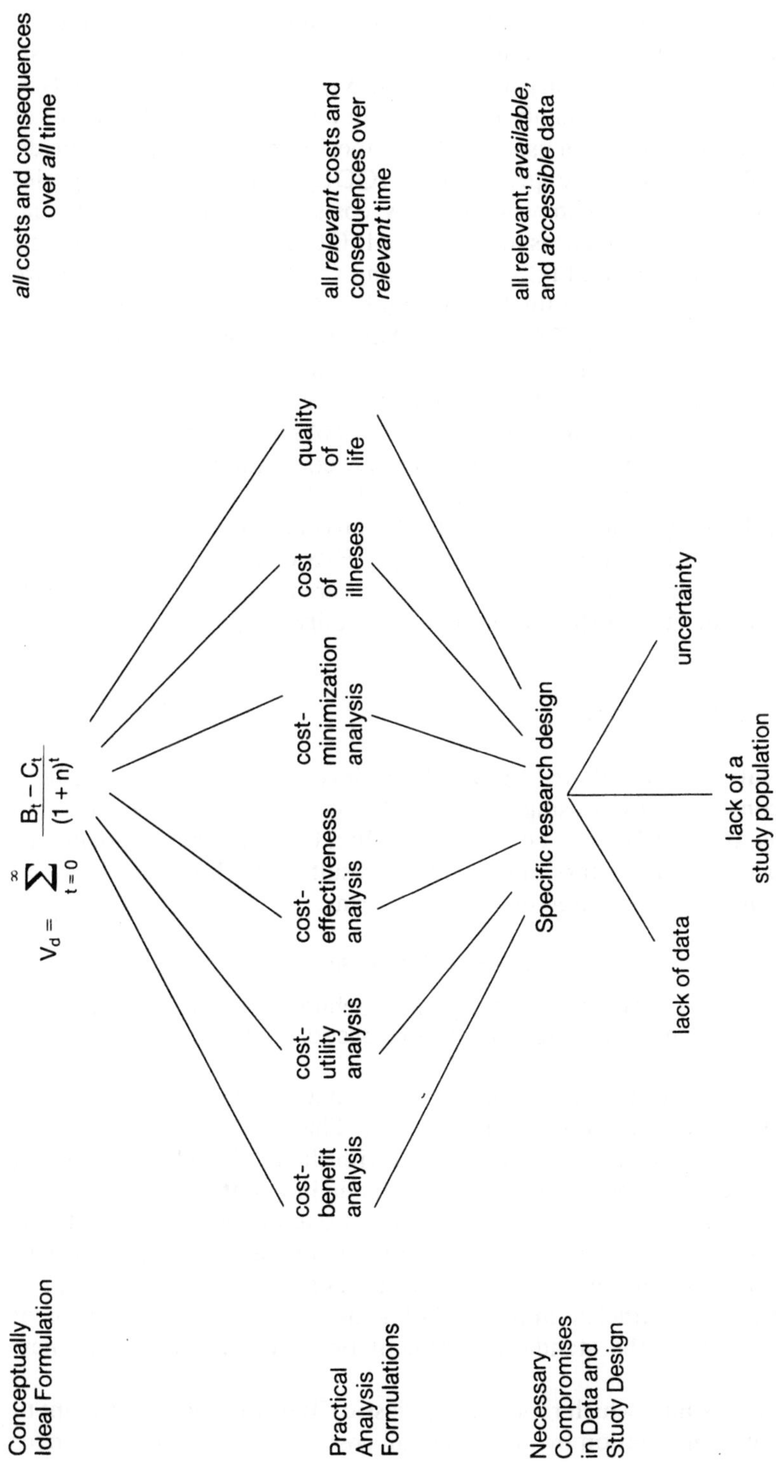

Fig. 3.1. Compromises in analysis from the ideal standard

is a specific research design that represents a compromise between the conceptual ideal and the constraints of working in an uncertain world of limited resources.

This book focuses on four different types of evaluations of medications: cost-benefit analysis (CBA), cost-utility analysis (CUA), cost-effectiveness analysis (CEA), and cost-minimization analysis (CMA). In addition, two other types of study are discussed that are often used for the socioeconomic evaluation of medications: cost-of-illness (COI) and quality of life (QOL) studies. These categories of evaluation differ primarily in whether only costs are measured (COI and CMA), whether only consequences are measured (QOL), or whether both costs and consequences are measured (CBA, CEA, and CUA). Studies that measure both costs and consequences are further distinguished by how consequences are measured: in economic terms (CBA), in natural units such as years of life (CEA), or in the utility or worth attributed to those natural units (CUA).

Although the terms "costs" and "consequences" are used in this book, not all texts use this terminology. For instance, reports of CBAs often discuss three types of outcomes: "costs" are the monetary inputs required to administer the technology or the program; "savings" are the resources that do not have to be used as a result of the technology; and "benefits" are the favorable outcomes, valued in monetary terms, that result from the technology. CEAs employ the terms "costs" and "savings" in the same sense; however, outcomes are measured in natural units of "effectiveness," most typically morbidity or mortality.

3.2.1 Cost-benefit Analysis

When the clinical outcomes of medications differ, it is necessary to examine both the costs and consequences of using the drugs. If consequences can be valued in economic terms, then a CBA can be performed. In a CBA all inputs and all outcomes are measured in monetary units, and the result is the difference between costs and consequences, measured in monetary terms.

Cost-benefit Analysis:

A socioeconomic analysis of any program or technology in which all real cost and consequences of that program are expressed in monetary terms.

In a CBA, both costs and consequences are monetary values; therefore, the result of a CBA is a net benefit for each treatment. This is important because the net benefits of one treatment can be compared with the net benefits of another, even though the treatment may be vastly different and have entirely different clinical outcomes. Because the result of a CBA is a net monetary benefit for the treatment, analysts may evaluate one treatment without comparing it explicitly with another. The reader should remember that, in studies having no explicit comparison, a comparison is nonetheless implicitly being made, either with a situation of "no treatment" or with the standard treatment prior to introducing the new technology.

In the following study, which represents a classic CBA, the authors attempt to approach the ideal formulation by measuring all costs and all consequences over all time in economic terms. This means that the authors must place a monetary value on saving lives, which is accomplished by using a proxy measure: the labor market value of individuals' work activity if they were healthy and able to work.

A Cost-Benefit Study: Rubella Vaccination

> This study examined the costs and consequences of providing rubella vaccination. The consequences were conceptualized as those costs that would be avoided with the vaccination program. Consequences included not only the averted medical costs associated with acute rubella and congenital rubella syndrome, but also the reduced economic productivity that results from disability or premature death. In order to place a monetary value on reduced productivity, the authors computed average lifetime earnings and estimated the amount of earnings that would be lost if no rubella vaccination program were in effect. They found that the costs of the program totaled \$28 937 400 and the value of lost productivity totaled \$9 521 200 for both medical conditions. (Schoenbaum et al. 1976 b)

There are a number of methods used to assign monetary values to human life but each has its drawbacks and the issue remains controversial. Criticisms of these methods are described in Chapter 5. Because of the problems inherent in placing monetary values on human life, many CBAs compromise on the ideal standard formulation. For example, in the following study no attempt was made to place a monetary value on the lives that were lost or saved. Instead total net medical care costs are reported separately and health outcomes are expressed in "natural units," that is, death rates. This formulation is similar to another type of study, the cost-effectiveness analysis, but, because the costs and the health consequences are reported separately rather in one equation, this is a CBA.

A Cost-Benefit Study: Pertussis Vaccination

> This study examined the cost-benefit of providing pertussis vaccination. Costs were measured as the resource cost of the vaccine, the treatment of complications resulting from the vaccine, and the treatment of cases of pertussis that resulted despite being vaccinated. These were called the costs with the program. Benefits were the savings in medical care costs by preventing pertussis and its sequelae. These were called the costs without the program. The benefit-cost ratio was:

$$\frac{\text{costs without program}}{\text{cost with program}}$$

or

$$\frac{\$1\,866\,153}{\$\ \ 720\,862} = 2.6:1$$

> This means that the benefits outweighed the costs by 2.6 times. The authors concluded that the pertussis vaccination program should be continued. Death rates under each scenario were reported separately. Under the worst case scenario, 6.3 people out of one million would die from the vaccination while 7.6 would die from pertussis if no vaccination were available. (Koplan et al. 1979)

It is very common for studies to report benefit-cost ratios; however, ratios can be misleading. Reporting net benefits rather than benefit-cost ratios is preferred for two reasons. First, ratios do not reveal which technology provides the largest absolute benefit, that is, projects or technologies with vastly different scales of costs may have similar ratios. For example, suppose one technology costs $2000 and results in $4000 worth of benefits while another costs $2 million and results in $3 million worth of benefits. The benefit-cost ratio for the first technology is 2 and for the second is 1.5. If we were to choose between the two technologies on the basis of the ratios we would choose the first technology, but the absolute value of the net benefits would be far greater from the second technology. Examining net benefits would lead to a more efficient choice.

The second reason that reporting net benefits is preferred to benefit-cost ratios concerns the ratio's sensitivity to how program effects are conceptualized. For example, say the cost of a technology is $1000 and the consequences fall into two categories: $500 savings in future medical costs and $1500 of direct health benefits. If medical cost savings were considered a "negative cost" rather than a benefit, then the following computations would result:
$1500 / ($1000−$500) = $1500/$500 = 3:1
benefit/(cost − "negative cost")

If medical cost savings were included as a benefit, then the following benefit-cost ratio would result:
($1500 + $500) / $1000 = $2000/$1000 = 2:1
(benefit + savings)/cost

No matter how net benefits are calculated, however, the results will be the same and policy decisions would be unchanged.
$1500 − ($1000−$500) = $1000
($1500 + $500) − $1000 = $1000

Thus far, we have examined a classic CBA that represents all costs and consequences in monetary terms, as well as a CBA that compromises on this ideal formulation by not placing a monetary value on human lives. What should be done when health effects data are not directly available? As an example the following study employed United States Medicaid claims data as a proxy for economic costs. This data base includes no information on health consequences. The two treatments are compared only with respect to their impact on health care expenditures with the implicit assumption that differences in health care costs reflect differences in health outcomes.

A Cost-Benefit Study: Cimetidine

In this study, the effects of cimetidine therapy were assessed in terms of financial outcomes. Information available in the Medicaid data base was used to control for patient characteristics and disease severity in the analysis. If these factors were not taken into account, then the differences in outcome between those patients who received cimetidine and those who were treated with conventional therapy may have resulted from differences in severity of illness.

> The authors found that patients who were treated with cimetidine experienced lower health care costs in their treatment for duodenal ulcer only if they had no health care expenditures during the previous year. If patients had high health care costs during the previous year, treatment with cimetidine during the study period was not associated with lower health care costs. (Geweke and Weisbrod 1982).

This study assumes that patients who use fewer medical services as a result of a particular treatment regimen are healthier. In other words, outcomes are not measured directly; rather, the savings in medical costs act as a proxy for measuring health consequences. It is assumed that patients who utilize fewer medical and surgical services to treat their ulcers are experiencing a positive health benefit that is reflected in lower resource use. For this assumption to be valid, any complications from the therapy or any treatment failure must have been treated using the Medicaid payment system. Alternatively, the reader must assume that, if non-Medicaid costs were considered, the conclusions drawn from the analysis would not differ substantially. In this particular study, it is probably valid to assume that decreased use of health services is a result of improved health status. For example, limited access to health care services does not appear to be a problem in this population, before or after treatment. The lesson here is that research reports must be read critically to determine whether implicit asumptions are indeed valid.

There are several disadvantages to using CBA for medical technologies.

1. A classic CBA formulation includes placing dollar values on outcomes that are not normally measured in strictly economic terms, for example, the value of a life.
2. If it seems impossible to place monetary values on consequences, then very important outcomes may simply be ignored in the analysis. Although this may occur with any difficult-to-measure consequences, it is more likely to happen when attempting to force noneconomic concepts into the economic mold.

3.2.2 Cost-utility Analysis

In cost-utility analysis (CUA), no attempt is made to measure health outcomes in monetary terms. Rather, CUA employs a common, nonmonetary metric to measure those consequences that are not amenable to economic expression. In CUA, outcomes are measured in terms of their quality or states of consumer preference. Several methods are available to estimate these "utility values" and will be discussed later in Chapter 12. Asking individuals to rate various health states is one method of assigning utility values.

Cost-utility Analysis:

> A socioeconomic evaluation that measures costs in monetary terms, but measures consequences in terms of their quality or "utility."

In a CUA, the cost of a treatment generally outweighs the savings that result from its use. When the analyst believes that economic costs are not a valid representation of the entire effects of a treatment and that decisions should not be based only on economic criteria, other important consequences of the use of a medication are measured. The outcomes that are measured in a CUA are years of life saved weighted or adjusted by their quality. This results in a measure called *quality-adjusted life years* or *QALYs*.

Cost-utility analysis represents a compromise from the ideal CBA in that some treatment outcomes are not measured in monetary terms; however, because not all outcomes are the same, this compromise still represents an improvement in our ability to measure health consequences.

A Cost-Utility Analysis: Pneumococcal Vaccine

This study examined the cost-utility of vaccination against pneumococcal pneumonia. Health outcomes were measured in quality-adjusted life years (QALYs). These calculations took into account the adverse effects of vaccination as well as the positive results of preventing pneumonia. Life years were weighted by the following values to "adjust" them for the quality of the health outcome:

0.0 = a year of death
0.4 = a year of disability in bed
0.6 = a year of disability out of bed
1.0 = a year of health

These values were obtained from a previous study that had asked respondents to rate various states of health. The authors reported results for different age groups that would hypothetically receive the vaccination.

Age when vaccinated	Cost per QALY
2– 4	\$77 200
5–24	\$55 300
25–44	\$22 900
45–64	\$ 5 700
>65	\$ 1 000

Because of the higher incidence of pneumonia among older individuals, cost-effectiveness increases with age. Thus, taking into account the differences in quality of life that might be achieved as well as the years of life saved, it is apparent that if any group is to be vaccinated it is the oldest age group.
(Willems et al. 1980)

The basic premise behind CUA is that all years of life saved are not necessarily equivalent. A year in the life of a cancer victim may be full of grief and pain and is certainly not equivalent to a year in the life of a patient with asymptomatic hypertension. However, the field of CUA is relatively new and the methods of obtaining utility values are being continually developed. Although theoretically, CUA appears to be a suitable method of comparing treatments to find the least costly way of obtaining a standard unit of health, its use is not always feasible. First, utility values have been developed for only a very narrow range of conditions. If established utility values are not available, values must be generated. This often entails interviews with patients and is not always feasible. Second, there is no consensus on how to obtain utility values and there is some discrepancy between values that are obtained by different methods.

3.2.3 Cost-effectiveness Analysis

In a CEA, inputs or costs are measured in monetary terms, but health outputs or consequences are measured in their natural units. Rather than attempting to place a monetary or utility value on health outputs, CEA employs measures such as years of life saved, or intermediate measures such as cases found, cases successfully treated, or cases averted. CEA is employed because of the difficulties inherent in measuring outcomes in CBA and CUA, and because CEA allows the assessment of intermediate outcomes. As with CUA, medical costs may outweigh the savings from treatment and it is necessary to measure noneconomic consequences in order more accurately to depict the true costs and effects of a treatment.

Cost-effectiveness Analysis:

A socioeconomic evaluation of two or more alternatives in which inputs are measured as economic costs but at least some outcomes are valued in non-monetary, but quantitative, terms.

In reporting the results of CEAs, many authors report cost-effectiveness ratios, that is, the average cost per unit of effectiveness (for example, dollars per life saved). These ratios can be misleading in CEAs just as in CBAs. Consider three treatments A, B, and C with the costs, effects, and cost-effectiveness ratios shown in Table 3.1.

Table 3.1. Comparing the cost-effectiveness of three treatments

Treatment	Cost	Effectiveness (number of cases prevented)	Cost-effectiveness ratio
A	$100000	12	8333
B	$200000	15	13333
C	$200000	12	16667

On the basis of these cost-effectiveness ratios, the program that required the smallest monetary investment for each case prevented would be chosen, that is, treatment A. But if we examine the situation a little more carefully we see that treatment B will prevent an additional three cases for $100000 more. This means that the cost for each additional case prevented would be $33333. The decision of whether these additional cases are worth $33 333 is a political and social decision, not a technical one. This information should be explicit in the report of the study, rather than remain hidden in the cost-effectiveness ratio.

A Cost-Effectiveness Study: Nicotine Gum

This study analyzed the cost-effectiveness of nicotine chewing gum in helping patients to stop smoking. The costs were measured as the cost of the gum and the amount of time physicians spend in prescribing it. The benefits were measure as the number of years of life saved for those who quit as a result of

> using the gum. Depending on the age and the sex of the patient, the costs of nicotine gum therapy were between $4113 and $9473 per year of life saved. (Oster et al. 1984)

One drawback of CEA is that consequences must be measured in identical units; that is, only interventions with the same outcome can be compared. For example, using CEA, a treatment whose primary outcome is to prevent allergy attacks cannot be compared with a treatment whose primary outcome is to reduce mortality from stroke.

Another drawback in using CEA is the implicit assumption that all outcomes, such as years of life saved, are equivalent. This means that adding 10 years to the life of a teenager is equivalent to adding 10 years to the life of an 80-year-old person and that an additional 10 years of life for one person are equivalent to adding 1 year of life for ten people. CUA may be a useful alternative in this situation.

3.2.4 Cost-minimization Analysis

The simplest type of socioeconomic analysis is the cost-minimization study (CMA). This type of study should be used only when it appears that treatments are identical in their effectiveness. Evidence for effectiveness is often provided from other studies such as randomized controlled trials. When such evidence is available, it is justifiable to compromise from the ideal CBA and examine only the costs of treatment.

Cost-Minimization Analysis:

> When two or more alternatives are shown to have equivalent clinical effectiveness, then only their net direct costs need be compared to identify the least costly alternative.

For two treatments to be equivalent means that the drugs must have precisely the same efficacy for all patients, under all conditions, with similar risks of adverse reactions. Such a remarkable degree of equivalence cannot often be assumed with certainty; therefore, cost-minimization analysis is relatively uncommon or it is performed improperly when true equivalence is not certain.

A Cost-Minimization Study: Intravenous Antibiotics

> This study compared several I, V, antibiotics. One of the antibiotics was administered once a day while the others were administered three or four times daily. Other studies had shown that the antibiotics were equal in effectiveness; therefore, this study examined only the differences in the costs of the drugs. To assess the costs of the drugs, only those cost data were collected that varied across the treatment regimens. These costs included: medications, supplies, administration and preparation time, and follow-up care. This study showed that using the once daily antibiotic resulted in savings of an average of $5.42 per patient per day, or between $23209 and $123243 per year for the hospital. (Eisenberg et al. 1984)

3.2.5 Cost of Illness Studies

Cost of illness studies may be thought of as precursors to socioeconomic evaluations of drugs. Rather than looking at the impact of treatments, cost of illness studies focus on the economic consequences of the medical conditions themselves. In essence, cost-of-illness studies illustrate the socioeconomic relevance of the disease or condition.

Cost of Illness Study:

A form of evaluation which computes the current economic impact of a disease, including the costs and consequences of treating that disease. No comparison of treatment modalities is involved.

The information provided by cost of illness studies is useful for two reasons:

1. It provides decision-makers with an estimate of the social impact of the disease to help them decide how best to allocate limited health care resources.
2. It can be incorporated into other studies like CEAs to show the economic benefits of treatments when illnesses are cured or prevented.

A Cost of Illness Study: Aminoglycoside-Induced Renal Failure

This study calculated the economic costs that result from kidney damage caused by aminoglycosides, a class of antibiotics. A group of patients who had received one of several aminoglycosides was examined. Those who suffered kidney damage were identified on the basis of laboratory tests of kidney function. The hospital costs incurred in caring for those with abnormal kidney function were compared with those patients who had normal test results. Costs were measured as additional days in the hospital, use of ancillary services, consultations with medical specialists, and use of the intensive care unit. Approximately 7% of the patients suffered kidney damage.

After controlling for severity of illness, it was found that patients who developed kidney damage had costs that were $2501 higher than those without this adverse effect. This meant that the average costs of kidney damage per patient treated with aminoglycosides was $183. For all patients treated with aminoglycosides during a 1-year period at this hospital, total costs of kidney damage were $321 348. This information could be used to assess the benefits of using an antibiotic that did not cause kidney damage. (Eisenberg et al. 1987)

Note that this study examined only the medical costs of illness; no attempt was made to measure health consequences suffered by the patient such as time lost from work or personal pain and suffering. Cost-of-illness studies may also include these nonmedical costs. When researchers measure the cost of an illness they face many of the same challenges inherent in CBA, CUA, and CEA. They must choose which costs are most relevant and how those costs will be valued. Thus, many of the compromises that must be made in other socioeconomic evaluations are faced in cost-of-illness studies as well. The principle of marginal analysis also applies to cost-of-illness studies. In some cases, analysts may be interested in the costs that could be saved if the disease were completely eradicated; however, eliminating

100% of the disease is likely to imply very high marginal costs in eliminating the final few cases.

One challenge that researchers face in estimating the cost of an illness is to avoid double-counting or undercounting. If all instances of a disease are counted regardless of whether that disease is listed as a primary or a secondary diagnosis, then the economic impact of a disease would be overestimated. The problem of undercounting arises when secondary diagnoses for certain diseases are disregarded. For example, diabetes mellitus is listed as a secondary diagnosis under cause of death three and a half times more often than it is listed as a primary cause of death (Jonsson 1983). When assessing a cost-of-illness study it is important to examine carefully how the researchers counted cases of morbidity and mortality, and to attempt to determine whether this could potentially under- or overestimate the cost of the disease.

3.2.6 Quality of Life Studies

Many clinical conditions, as well as medical interventions such as drugs and surgery, potentially have impact on the quality of patients' lives. There are presently available a number of methods that can be used to evaluate the total physical, psychological, and social well-being of a person. It is possible not only to base treatment decisions on the biomedical efficacy of a medication, but also to consider the effects of the medication on a broad spectrum of indicators of a patient's quality of life.

Quality of Life Study:

The evaluation of the impact of a disease or a medical service on the social, physiological, mental, intellectual, and general well-being of individuals.

Social functioning is measured as the ability of individuals to fullfill their social roles, that is, how well do people do what is expected of them by others? It includes the ability to work, to fulfill responsibilities in the family, and to interact meaningfully with friends and as a member of the community. Physical functioning includes activities of daily living such as being able to dress oneself and being mobile. It also includes physical symptoms such as pain and nausea. Emotional functioning is measured by asking people about their feelings. Are they depressed? Do they have anxiety? Do they feel they can cope with pressures? Intellectual functioning includes memory, alertness, the ability to learn and make decisions, and the ability to organize and complete tasks. Finally, general well-being includes a wide variety of dimensions such as satisfaction with life and spiritual well-being.

Quality of life is usually measured using a questionnaire or interview format. Scales (lists of questions with standardized answers) have been developed that measure quality of life across many different types of people with varying clinical conditions. Chapter 10 contains a more detailed explanation of the concept of quality of life and its assessment as well examples of questions that are used to measure quality of life.

Although considerable work has been done in refining the concept of quality of life and in devising instruments that measure quality of life, this area of research is still in its early stages. There is no current consensus on how to conceptualize quality of life, how best to measure its components, or how the components interact with one another. Nevertheless, instruments are being developed that have a high degree of psychometric validity and the importance of the area is unquestioned.

A Quality of Life Study: Auranofin Therapy

In this randomized double-blind clinical trial, auranofin (oral gold) was compared with placebo in therapy for patients with rheumatoid arthritis. In addition to standard clinical measures of treatment response (number of tender or swollen joints, grip strength, stiffness and walking time), 19 other outcome measures were obtained. These included assessments of: daily functioning and activity, range of motion tasks, mobility, physical activity, social activity, detailed patient assessments of pain, global assesment of arthritis, and global assessment of overall health.

The results of this study showed that patients treated with auranofin scored consistently higher on these quality of life measures than patients who continued normal therapy. (Bombardier et al. 1986)

It is possible to obtain quality of life information not only from patients but from clinicians and patients' family members. As this next study shows, the results can sometimes be very different depending on the source of the information.

A Quality of Life Study: Effects of Antihypertensive Medication

Seventy-five hypertensive patients were asked to evaluate their quality of life since beginning medication to lower their blood pressure. In addition, their clinicians and a family member were also requested to rate patients' quality of life. Questions were asked regarding impairments in memory, worry, irritability, mood, interest in life, initiative, energy, activity, hypochondria, and sexual function. Patients were on a variety of medications: beta-blockers, diuretics, methyldopa, and combination therapies.

Physicians reported that all patients were improved since beginning antihypertensive therapy; however, only 48% of patients reported improvement in any of the areas, while 8% reported some decline in quality of life. Only one family member reported that the patient had improved since beginning therapy. The most commonly reported quality of life areas which were adversely affected were energy, mood, activity, and hypochondria. (Jachuk et al. 1982).

Quality of life studies provide explicit information about how a treatment affects a wide array of important personal and social areas of functioning. CUA and CEA both attempt to measure health consequences of treatments in non-monetary terms. Both methods provide a summary measure of health effects: CEA in natural units and CUA in utilities. These methods are extremely useful in that they provide a single index of costs versus consequences; however, reducing such complex concepts into a single measure results in a simplification of reality that may be too great. We may know that, with CUA, a certain change in quality-adjusted life years is associated with a certain level of investment in medical resources, but what is the nature of that "quality?" We may be able to compare several treatments in a succinct fashion using CEA and CUA, but it is not possible to describe in detail the types of health effects that result from a treatment. Quality of life studies compromise between the greater richness of data they provide and the less concise nature of the output. On the other hand, QALYs embody explicit information about the weights attached to different components of the quality of life and this information is not given in quality of life descriptions alone. An ideal QALY study will provide both the descriptive detail and the summary statistic embodying the weighted components. It is an ideal worth striving for.

3.2.7 Budgetary Analysis

Another form of socioeconomic evaluation is the *budgetary analysis* that assesses the impact of a certain program or technology on the budget of a specific agency or institution. A governmental agency in charge of making decisions about the introduction of a new drug into the nation's health care system may wish to examine the impact of that drug on its health care expenditures. A hospital wishing to make a decision about accepting a new drug on its formulary may also conduct a budgetary analysis. In both cases, the study has very specific boundaries and examines a very restricted range of costs and consequences, namely those which pertain only to the welfare of the agency, not the welfare of society in general.

As an example, a study may be conducted that examines the impact of introducing a new medication on the drug budget of a nation. The study may be conducted in a technically sound manner, adhering to the quidelines proposed in this book; however, policy decisions emanating from the study will be less than optimal because of the restricted focus of the analysis. The study may examine only those expenditures for which the agency is responsible and may not assess the savings in future medical costs or improvements in economic productivity of patients receiving the drug. The study will not therefore provide an examination of the true socioeconomic impact of the medication. It may overestimate or underestimate the costs and consequences associated with introducing the drug. Decision-makers whose charge is to make decisions for the good of society will be misled by the results of such a study. This topic is considered further under "Perspective" in Chapter 4.

Conclusion

We have discussed several analytical formulations that may be employed to study the socioeconomic impact of drugs. The specific formulation used in a study depends on the problem to be analyzed, the data that are available, and the valuation methods that will be used. One type of socioeconomic evaluation is not inherently better or worse than another. However, in any particular case, one method is likely to be more appropriate than another based on the types of question asked and the types of data that are available.

Cost-benefit analyses value health outcomes in monetary terms. Cost-utility analyses weight health outcomes to account for the differences between outcomes that are not captured by traditional morbidity and mortality measures. Cost-effectiveness analyses express consequences in terms of morbidity and mortality, but can also assess cost per case detected or cost per case prevented. Cost-minimization analyses concentrate on the health care costs associated with interventions. Cost-of-illness studies estimate the total economic impact of a disease or a condition. Quality of life studies measure the impact of conditions or treatments on the total personal and social well-being of patients. Each of these forms of analysis attempts to measure the social and economic impact of diseases or their treatments. They step beyond an assessment of the clinical efficacy of a medication and attempt to understand the effects of treatments in a much broader sense.

Through socioeconomic evaluations it is possible to make better informed decisions regarding the use, distribution, and financing of medications. Decisions regarding the adoption of a medication are often based on a simple budgetary analysis that asks: what is the unit cost of this medication? What is the prevalence of the disease? The product of these numbers then represents the cost of this medication to the hospital's drug budget or the drug budget of the nation. Full-scale socioeconomic evaluations are preferable to this limited budgetary analysis because they highlight the vast array of costs and consequences that should be considered in making a judgment regarding the adoption of medications. These costs and consequences provide a much richer base of information for decision-makers, allowing them to understand the varied effects of a medication and those costs that are often hidden.

4 Framework of the Evaluation

4.1 Introduction

In this chapter, we begin to outline certain standards that are expected of all socioeconomic evaluations, regardless of the study type. As discussed in Chap. 3, a socioeconomic evaluation ideally examines all benefits and all costs that accrue to all people over all time relative to all possible alternatives. However, because resources are limited, it is necessary to compromise and to restrict the framework of the evaluation. The focus of a study should be explicitly defined early in a study report, and the first step in defining the focus is the research question. Following a discussion of the elements of the research question, this chapter concludes with a discussion of the pathways of clinical management.

4.2 Defining the Research Question

Vital to understanding any socioeconomic evaluation is a clear understanding of the research question that is addressed in the study. The research question is defined by stating

1. the objectives of the analysis,
2. the perspective taken, and
3. the alternatives considered.

Early in the course of a study report, the reader should be able to identify the precise problem that is being addressed.

> "The objective of our study was to assess the economic and health consequences of various expensive antimicrobial regimens in seriously ill patients." (Weinstein et al. 1986)

> "The purpose of this article is to present a recalculation of the benefits, risks, and costs of pertussis and pertussis vaccine, using recently published information." (Hinman and Koplan 1984)

From these problem statements, the following information can be gleaned:
a) a general idea of the clinical condition and patient population of interest,
b) the type of drug therapy or therapies analyzed, and (c) the range of inputs and outcomes analyzed.

The research question or problem statement thus sets the stage for the remainder of the analysis. The perspective, the alternatives under comparison, and the clinical management pathways flow naturally from these stated objectives.

4.3 The Perspective

The perspective of the study refers to the viewpoint from which the analysis is performed. Typically, four major viewpoints can be taken, those of:
1. Society
2. Third party payers (including government, health insurance companies, and health maintenance organizations)
3. The health provider (the clinic, hospital, and clinicians)
4. Patients.

From each viewpoint there are different information needs and different criteria of evaluation. Perspective is important for making decisions regarding the use of the medication. What is cost-effective for one party (for example, the hospital) may not be cost-effective for another (for example, a third party payer). Costs and consequences that are relevant to one party may be irrelevant to another.

Perspective:

The viewpoint from which the analysis is conducted. A determinant of the types of cost and consequence that will be examined and the conclusions that can be drawn from the study. Ideally, socioeconomic evaluations should be performed from the perspective of society if the results are to be used for societal-level resource allocation decisions.

4.3.1 The Perspective of Society

A newly introduced medication should improve social welfare in general. Thus, the ideal evaluation takes the perspective of society. A societal perspective should examine the entire social and economic effect of the technology on all segments of society. This might entail scrutiny of a wide array of health consequences and economic costs incurred in hospital care, outpatient care, long-term care, home care, and social welfare services regardless of when they are incurred or who must pay for them. In addition, a broad range of other social, ethical, and legal consequences might be examined. Such a study is termed technology assessment.

Technology assessment:

An evaluation of the impact of a technology on a broad array of costs and consequences including some that cannot be quantified. The aim of technology assessment is to identify potentially hidden costs and consequences which, if known, may change resource allocation decisions.

Although all technologies do not warrant such a comprehensive "ideal" examination, technologies that are extremely expensive, that may have the capability to shift relatively large amounts of resources from one sector of the economy to another, or that may raise other major social concerns deserve such investigation. Heart transplantation is an example of one technology that has received such a thorough analysis.

A Comprehensive Study from the Societal Perspective

> The National Heart Transplantation Study was funded by the Health Care Financing Administration of the United States government. The purpose of the study was to explore all ramifications of heart transplantation technology. The following issues were examined in this five-volume report:
> 1. Need for heart transplantation, thus estimating the probable volume of transplants
> 2. Availability of organs
> 3. Diffusion of transplant technology
> 4. Quality of life for organ transplant recipients
> 5. Economic costs of heart transplantation
> 6. Sources of payment for the technology
> 7. Ethical issues such as recipient selection, definition of death of the donor, and ethical allocation of transplant resources
> 8. Legal issues relating to donors and recipients, as well as regulation of transplant services such as certification of providers and antitrust laws
> 9. Analysis of a potential alternative to heart transplantation: the artificial heart. (Evans et al. 1984)

Notwithstanding the value of the comprehensive societal perspective, most evaluations of medications taking the social point of view are usually limited to analyzing a narrover range of consequences that can be attributed directly to the use of the drug. The reader should be aware of the more limited nature of this common form of evaluation and should evaluate whether important social, legal, and ethical consequences are being ignored.

A Narrower Study from a Societal Perspective

> This study examined the cost-effectiveness of cholestyramine therapy as a preventive measure against heart disease. By including the net social costs (of which medical costs were but one component) and the net increase in life expectancy, a societal perspective was taken.
> The societal costs and consequences that were examined included lifetime medical costs associated with decreased incidence of cardiac disease, the costs of treating noncardiac illness in the added years of life attributable to hyperlipemic therapy, and the years of life saved as a result of therapy. (Oster and Epstein 1987)

Although the societal perspective is the ideal way of determining the value of a drug and only this perspective considers all potential costs and consequences, many studies are performed from the more limited perspectives of the third party payer and the provider. It is very important to realize that such studies will not necessarily lead to conclusions that are optimal for society as a whole. For example, studies performed from a limited perspective may lead to resource allocation decisions that will result in inefficient cost-shifting from one budget to another. If a more limited perspective is taken, it should be limited in a way that has been fully discussed with the customer for the study (if the customer can be readily identified) and the analyst should report exactly what potential costs and consequences are excluded from the study so that the reader (and customer) should beware of the incomplete nature of the analysis (Akehurst and Buxton 1985). Thus, the first level of compromise in defining the framework for the evaluation is often to narrow the societal perspective to the most relevant social costs and consequences. A second-order compromise is to take a narrower perspective such as those described in the next sections.

4.3.2 The Perspective of the Third Party Payer

The third party payer may be private insurance companies, health maintenance organizations, or the government. The third party payer will be primarily interested in the costs of reimbursing health care providers for their services. Their first concern is the efficiency of that portion of the health care delivery system for which they reimburse medical services; therefore an analysis from this perspective must ideally capture the entire stream of medical care expenses incurred or avoided due to the new technology. The expenses of interest are mainly those for which the third party payer is responsible. Therefore, expenses such as patient out-of-pocket payments, or costs such as lost productivity attributable to disability, are technically irrelevant from the viewpoint of the third party payer, although these may be significant costs from the perspective of society.

A Study from the Viewpoint of a Third Party Payer

In an evaluation of the economic effects of cimetidine compared with routine therapy for duodenal ulcers, the perspective of a public insurer (Medicaid) was taken. For this study, Medicaid claims records were used as the source of data; therefore only Medicaid expenditures were examined. This study did not include costs that accrued to other insurers, providers, or patients. In addition, noneconomic benefits were also not considered. (Geweke and Weisbrod 1982)

In this study, a compromise was made between a full societal evaluation and the constraints under which the researchers worked. Ideally, the drug should have been evaluated from the perspective of society in order to trace the broadest array of costs and benefits across the widest spectrum of patients. However, the realities of data availability and the need to assess an important medication on a limited research budget led the researchers to choose this perspective. Because the authors explicitly described the perspective of their analysis, the reader is forewarned about the limitations of the study and can take these limitations into account in interpreting the results.

4.3.3 The Perspective of the Health Care Provider

Health care providers include hospitals, clinics, and clinicians. From the hospital and clinic perspective, those costs which influence the expenses of providing health care in their particular institution will be most important. Thus, the provider's perspective is narrower than that of the insurer.

A Study from the Provider's Viewpoint

> This study compared the costs of outpatient versus inpatient cancer chemotherapy. The two treatment methods were considered to have the same efficacy. The costs which were examined included only those costs borne by the hospital and the outpatient clinic. In drawing conclusions about the study's results, the authors specifically addressed the needs of hospital administrators and physicians who are attempting to reduce their costs of providing medical care. (Wodinsky et al. 1987)

In the example cited above, it is likely that the narrower perspective taken by the analysts is appropriate because there are no obvious inefficiencies or other consequences that involve nonhospital resources. In this case, the perspective of the health care provider may coincide with the broader social perspective.

If some complications of therapy are possible after the initial hospitalization, a narrow provider perspective would clearly be inappropriate. Although a patient could be "successfully" treated during the course of therapy, a treatment complication could very well occur later and might require a subsequent hospitalization, perhaps at a different institution. Although the treatment may be cost-effective from the perspective of the hospital that initially treated the patient, subsequent morbidity and rehospitalization can render the initial treatment inefficient, that is, not cost-effective from the perspective of society (or, for that matter, from the perspective of the third party payer or the patient).

4.3.4 The Patient's Perspective

From the viewpoint of the patient, costs that affect out-of-pocket payments will be most consequential, while costs borne by others will count little. For example, a medication that enables patients to be treated outside the hospital may represent higher out-of-pocket expenditures to the patient. While early discharge from the hospital will result in savings for the hospital, shifting care from an institutional to an outpatient setting, where medications are not reimbursed by insurance, may result in higher costs for the patient. Other issues of importance to the patient are quality of life, time lost from work, and the need for child care or housekeeping services while receiving medical care. These costs are also considered from the societal perspective. Although few studies are conducted from the patient perspective, this discussion outlines patient costs and consequences which should be incorporated in studies conducted from the societal point of view.

A Study from the Perspective of the Patient

This study examined the costs of rheumatoid arthritis therapy by asking patients about the economic and personal costs associated with the condition. Economic costs included hospital care, physician and therapist visits, laboratory and radiological testing, the purchase of devices, and the use of nontraditional therapies such as acupuncture. In addition, the patients completed questionnaires that assessed the disability resulting from arthritis and its impact on their general health. (Lubeck et al. 1986)

4.3.5 Perspective: An Overview

Perspective is a key element in defining the research question and in governing which costs and consequences will be of interest and how they will be analyzed. Ideally, relevant costs and consequences are examined from the perspective of society. This dictates that costs and consequences be included regardless of who experiences them. The perspective of the third party payer and, to a lesser extent, that of a providing institution is commonly found in the literature. The reader should ask whether such an orientation compromises key elements that might be included from a societal perspective and, thus, leads to incorrect conclusions regarding resource allocation. Analyses conducted from the perspective of the patient or the physician are uncommon. Regardless of what perspective is taken, the choice should be clearly stated in the research report and limitations should be identified.

4.4 The Alternatives

It is hard to overstate the importance of the alternative interventions being compared because the choice of alternatives can govern whether or not an analysis will demonstrate cost-effectiveness for a particular treatment. Socioeconomic evaluations are inherently comparative, asking "cost-effective compared with what?" The answer should normally be, "compared with the course of therapy that would otherwise be used for the decision being examined," or "compared with another therapy that is a candidate for patients of this type."

Alternatives:

The options which are examined in a socioeconomic evaluation; alternatives should reflect practical choices that clinicians encounter.

The issue of choosing alternatives is closely intertwined with that of perspective. For example, consider a study conducted to provide information about a new blood pressure medication for a reimbursement or formulary decision. From the limited perspective of a hospital formulary or a nation's drug budget, the alternative would be another drug that would potentially be replaced. However, from the social perspective or from the point of view of an organized health care system interested in the most efficient treatment regardless of modality, the alternative might well be an educational program aimed at restricting sodium in the diet. It is critical to realize that every socioeconomic evaluation is necessarily a comparison of at least two alternatives.

The alternatives include: a) no treatment, b) placebo, c) another medication, d) surgery, e) behavioral or lifestyle changes.

No Treatment as the Alternative

> This study examined the cost-effectiveness of screening and immunizing pregnant women for hepatitis B. The treatment options were screening with subsequent immunization of positive cases versus not screening. (Arevalo and Washington 1988)

The alternatives being compared should be described in sufficient detail that it is possible to understand what the alternatives are, how they were administered, and how patients were assigned to receive them.

Placebo as the Alternative

> This study compared oral gold therapy with placebo to assess the cost-effectiveness of oral gold. Information was obtained on quality of life as well as costs of therapy. Placebo patients received the normal course of therapy that would be expected in actual clinical practice. (Thompson et al. 1988)

Although the administration of a placebo is not considered a viable option in clinical practice, data on placebo may often be the only ones available on a medication's efficacy because informations is obtained from a clinical trial that compared the medication with placebo. When placebo is the alternative, it can be assumed that the alternative is either the no therapy option or standard therapy, depending upon the description of the alternative in the study report. In addition, for some analyses, the alternative may not be explicity stated, in which case the alternative is "no treatment".

Surgical Therapy as the Alternative

> Two major treatment alternatives for prostatic cancer are estrogen therapy and orchiectomy (surgical castration). This study examined the cost-effectiveness of these alternatives. Estrogen therapy consisted of monthly injections of medication plus oral estrogen. In addition, estrogen-treated patients underwent one X-ray treatment of the breasts to prevent breast enlargement. Patients who received orchiectomy had one operation under general anesthesia. (Hendriksson and Edhag 1987)

When the medication is compared with a surgical procedure, another medication, or a change in behavior or life-style, it must be realized that the treatments are not always mutually exclusive. For example, in the treatment of open-angle glaucoma, it is possible to use surgery or beta-blocking drugs. Patients started on the medication may become refractory to drug treatment, in which case the eventual therapy will be surgery. The scenario described in a study should ideally include the possibility of this change in treatment and the study design should be constructed to allow for analysis of changes in therapy (Dao 1985).

Another Medication as an Alternative

Three different treatments aimed at lowering blood cholesterol levels were compared: cholestyramine, cholestipol, and oat bran. A wide range of costs were computed, including those which were similar across the medications tested. Therefore, an implicit alternative of no therapy was also being considered. (Kinosian and Eisenberg 1988)

When the reader evaluates the study report, one question that should arise is whether the alternatives presented are the most appropriate ones. First, are the alternatives being compared actually the alternatives that are available in realistic settings? Second, are the alternatives relevant for the particular policy decision under consideration? That is, do they address the interests of the party from whose perspective the study is conducted?

Behavior Change as an Alternative

Two medications prescribed for weight loss were compared with a placebo condition and with behavioral therapy in order to assess the relative cost-effectiveness of each treatment form. Behavior therapy consisted of a program of behavior modification aimed at changing eating and exercise patterns. (Dahms et al. 1978)

4.4.1 The Research Question: An Overview

Thus far, this chapter has examined the research question and its components. Study reports should explicitly state the objective of the study, the perspectives from which the study is performed, and the alternatives with which the technology of interest is being compared. The objectives, the perspective, and the alternatives will determine to a large extent whether the study is appropriate for the reader's decision-making needs and whether the drug of interest will prove to be cost-effective. Essentially, once the research question has been stated, the reader should be aware of the initial assumptions made by the researchers. Understanding these assumptions will allow the reader to judge the relevance and the validity of the study results.

4.5 Pathways of Clinical Management

An important part of structuring a socioeconomic evaluation is to explicate the pathways of clinical management. This entails outlining: a) the resources that are required to provide a service, b) how the resources are combined and c) what possible outcomes might be expected from that combination of resources.

This is, in essence, a description of the clinical production relationship. It is the responsibility of the analyst to specify clearly the clinical management pathway employed in an evaluation. This description allows the reader to understand what costs and consequences were considered in the analysis.

Pathway of Clinical Management:

A description or model that describes the process of diagnosis and treatment, including expected patterns of resource utilization and possible outcomes after the intervention.

There are alternative means of treating health problems and each results in a different clinical pathway. Alternative diagnostic modalities can substitute for one another. Drugs may be used instead of surgery. Conditions may be treated on an inpatient or an outpatient basis. The stream of clinical events that culminates in a health outcome will change in response to the introduction of new diagnostic and treatment methods.

The construction of clinical management pathways is linked to the research question in that the medical intervention that is being assessed can be delivered in either an "ideal" fashion or a somewhat less-than-ideal fashion. For instance, a cost-effectiveness analysis of blood pressure medication versus a diet and exercise program can be depicted in an ideal setting where drug levels are perfectly maintained, patient compliance is assured, and medical follow-up is thorough. Such an analysis depicts the *efficacy* of the drug, that is, how well it performs under ideal conditions. On the other hand, the drug can be analyzed within a typical community setting, where there may be poor drug control, erratic patient compliance, and sporadic follow-up. This analysis depicts the *effectiveness* of the medication, that is, how well it works under more typical conditions. The pathways of clinical management for these two scenarios will be very different from one another and this difference can have an enormous impact on the results of the analysis. A statement of the research objectives should describe whether the technology is being analyzed under ideal or routine conditions.

Ideally, the alternative pathways of clinical management are clearly stated and unambiguous; however, this is not typically the case in most research reports. Because the production of health is not always clearly understood even by health care practitioners, it is not always possible to describe the production process. There is also considerable diversity in the practice of medicine across physicians and regions (Wennberg et al. 1987). Thus precise and unambiguous descriptions of management pathways that account for a broad range of practitioners and practice styles may not even be possible.

Rather than presenting explicit pathways of clinical management, most authors compromise by simply listing the inputs and the outputs in a production process and provide less information on how resources are combined to achieve the outcomes. As a result, it may be difficult to discern whether the resources were used efficiently, whether they were combined in the most suitable proportions, or whether all the inputs were actually necessary to achieve the output.

In light of this limitation, it is necessary for the reader to examine the clinical management pathways critically for the treatment alternatives being compared. The reader should postulate what additional resources might be required, what further treatment steps might lead from the course of action described, and whether the resource use described in the study differs significantly from that in actual practice. Only by understanding the clinical management pathways can the reader evaluate whether the costs and the consequences of the alternatives analyzed in the study are appropriate and whether the results presented are relevant to their own decision-making needs.

Even though fully explicated management pathways cannot be expected in every research report, the author is obliged to make at least two things very clear. First, the research report should state whether the resource use described in the study report represents an ideal scenario or clinical practice under normal operating conditions. Second, the report should provide a detailed listing of precisely which costs and consequences were included in the analysis and which were omitted together with the grounds for inclusion or exclusion.

An Example of a Clinical Production Relationship

The costs and outcomes associated with pertussis and pertussis vaccine were assessed by estimating the rates of illness without the vaccine, the rates of complications and prevention of pertussis with the vaccine, and the expected expenditures with and without the vaccine. The authors based their figures on recent clinical studies. They tried to estimate all the medical costs and outcomes that would occur in two scenarios: one with a vaccine program and one without. They estimated:

1. Rates of hospitalization, death, and encephalitis that would result from pertussis
2. Rates of adverse reactions attributable to pertussis vaccination
3. Expected costs of physician visits, hospitalizations, length of stay, and long-term care resulting from pertussis infection
4. Expected costs of medical resource use to treat reactions to the vaccine
5. Vaccine cost

By enumerating these possible costs and outcomes, this study defined a large part of the production relationship. (Hinman and Koplan 1984)

Many authors choose to illustrate pathways of clinical management using models that depict graphically how patients are treated, what the expected outcomes are from each treatment, what expected patterns of resource utilization occur after the treatments, and what clinical outcomes might be expected as a result of each intervention.

Figure 4.1 is an example of a pathway of clinical management for treatment of gonorrhea. Note that patients receive one of three treatment alternatives: tetracycline, ampicillin, or a combination therapy. Possible treatment and health outcomes are described in separate tree diagrams. The utilization of medical services is implicit in these descriptions of cure and pregnancy outcomes. The reader should note that graphic depictions of decision trees inevitably require simplification of the actual medical process and, by simplifying, we necessarily compromise between ease of depiction and the richness and complexity of clinical reality. The question is, as always, whether these compromises are warranted given the issue at hand, a question that a good study will address explicitly.

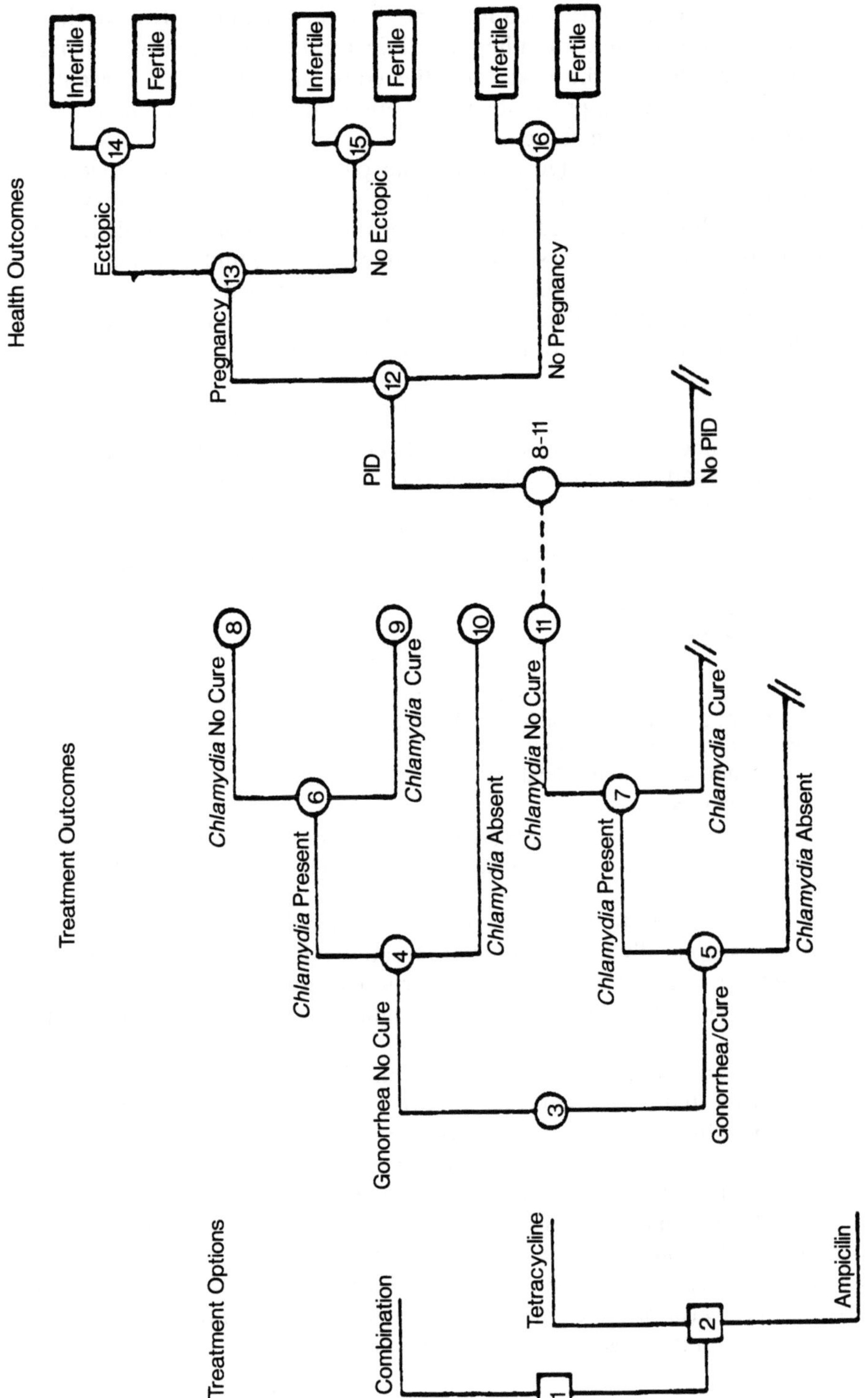

Fig. 4.1. Pathway of clinical management for treatment of gonorrhea. (Washington et al. 1987)

4.6 Conclusion

This chapter described the study framework, the research question, and pathways of clinical management. The research question states the objective of the research and is the foundation for the alternatives, perspectives, and, ultimately, the pathway of clinical management that will be considered in the study. The perspective defines, to a large extent, the types of cost and consequence that will be assessed and is a powerful determinant of the conclusions that will be drawn from the study results. Generally, the societal perspective is preferred because it considers the general social welfare rather than only the viewpoint of a specific player.

Socioeconomic evaluations, by definition, compare one treatment with another, even if the comparison is "no treatment." The demonstration of cost-effectiveness depends to a large extent on the alternatives analyzed; thus, the study report should justify why specific alternatives were chosen. Furthermore, these alternatives should represent real clinical choices.

Finally, a study report should describe the pathways of clinical management, or at least the inputs and outputs that are examined in a study. Enough information should be presented so that the reader is able to identify those significant costs and consequences that were not assessed. Compromises are often necessary in structuring an analysis, but the evaluation report should state explicitly what compromises were made and whether this limits the applicability of the study results.

5 Assessing Costs

5.1 Introduction

The practice of socioeconomic evaluation is limited by the state of knowledge about a particular area and the state of data availability. Nowhere is this more apparent than in the assessment of costs. While the process of identifying resources and assigning monetary costs may seem relatively straightforward, there are numerous problems that confront researchers during this process. The identification of costs and the problems that can arise are the subjects of this chapter.

The economic aspects of a medical intervention flow essentially in parallel with its clinical aspects. Thus, one can imagine two parallel streams in the treatment of a disease: a clinical and an econonmic stream (see Fig. 5.1). Events in one stream will have a direct counterpart in the other; each stage of the clinical management of a patient is associated with economic costs. Diagnosis, treatment, and the management of sequelae and side effects can all be examined not only in terms of the medical process but also in terms of medical resource consumption or economics.

If clinical events can be characterized in terms of their economic consequences, then each clinical event is potentially expressible as a monetary value. Every addi-

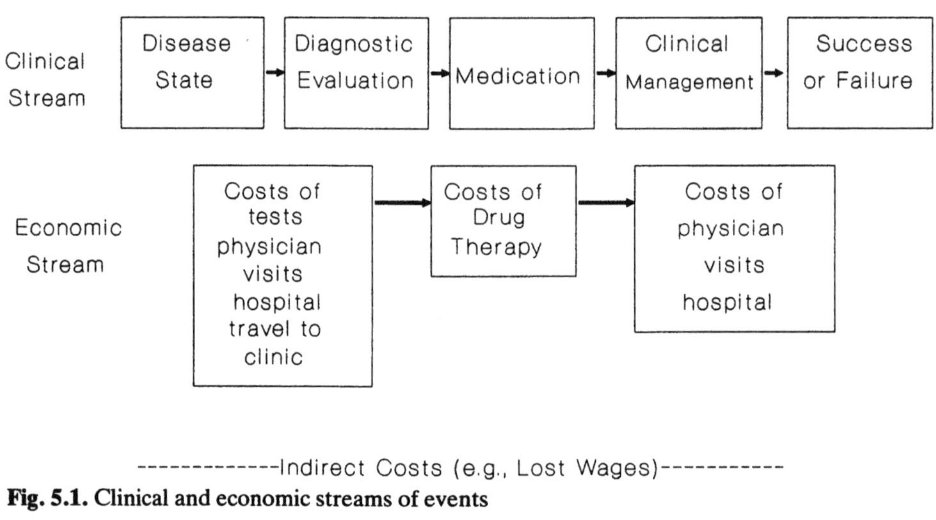

Fig. 5.1. Clinical and economic streams of events

tional diagnostic test, each additional day in the hospital, and each clinic visit has an associated economic worth. An episode of medical care which is efficient in terms of its use of medical resources will also be *clinically efficient* if we trace the entire stream of events and if the episode is examined from the societal perspective. Skimping on medical services during a particular hospitalization may be economically efficient over the short run and from the viewpoint of the hospital; however, subsequent medical problems, rehospitalization, and loss of patient productivity reveal the clinical inefficiency of this course of therapy.

As described in Chapter 2, researchers would ideally like to identify the opportunity costs of alternative treatments or the value of alternatives that are forgone. However, estimating this opportunity cost is often difficult. The process would ideally entail enumerating all resources that are expended in pursuing a certain alternative. Some of these resources are obvious and easily estimated while others, such as volunteer time and the value of patients' time, are less apparent and not always easily quantifiable. The researcher inevitably engages in a series of compromises between this ideal and the reality of measuring resource use and determining monetary costs.

This chapter will provide the background for determining whether the appropriate resources were identified and whether they were estimated or valued correctly. It will provide the reader with an understanding of the difference between direct and indirect costs, variable and fixed costs, and medical and nonmedical costs. Later in the chapter, various nuances of costing that are specific to socioeconomic studies are discussed. This is an important chapter because costing tends to be much more complex than is often realized. In fact, the literature is rife with otherwise sound scientific articles that contain incomplete or erroneous costing analyses.

5.2 Types of Costs

There are two general categories of costs: direct costs and indirect costs. *Direct costs* include actual changes in resource use that are attributable to the medication. It is important to examine not only those direct medical costs that are associated with the drug, but to look beyond drug costs to other sectors of the health care market.

Direct Costs:

Changes in resource utilization that are required for or attributable to the intervention being studied. Includes both medical and nonmedical components.

Direct Costs

A cost-effectiveness study of the treatment of tuberculosis included the following direct costs.

1. Costs of the medications
2. Costs of diagnostic tests: tuberculin tests, sputum cultures, chest Xray, drug susceptibility screening, complete blood counts

3. Costs of adverse reactions to the medications, such as hepatitis and gastro-intestinal upset. These costs included physician office visits, laboratory test, and hospitalization.

This study included not only the direct costs of the medication, but also the costs of diagnosing tuberculosis and treating side effects of the medications. (Snider et al. 1986)

Direct nonmedical costs should ideally also be incorporated into the analysis. These include resource expenditures outside the medical care market, such as costs borne by patients in seeking care.

Direct Nonmedical Costs

In a study examining outpatient intravenous antibiotic therapy for patients with osteomyelitis, the following nonmedical inputs were incorporated into the analysis:

1. Patient transportation to and from hospital
2. Extra trips to the emergency room
3. Child care expenses
4. Housekeeping costs. (Eisenberg and Kitz 1986)

Direct costs are subdivided into *fixed* and *variable* costs. Variable costs vary with the volume of services rendered while fixed costs remain constant across the entire range of service volumes. It is important to differentiate between fixed and variable costs, particularly when examining changes in the volume of services as a means of improving cost-effectiveness.

By definition, variable costs such as medical supplies or medications are gained or lost depending on whether they are used and in what volumes. On the other hand, fixed costs are "fixed", that is, they cannot be "saved", at least in the short run, regardless of whether or not they are used. Thus "saving" a hospital day will results in saving variable costs such as supplies and medications, but will not save fixed costs, such as administration costs, debt, and other overheads.

What about nursing hours that are saved? Do they represent a fixed or a variable cost? Clearly the *hours* are "saved" in that they are not allocated to the patients who were discharged early. But can the hospital administrator count on "saving" the dollars that those hours represent? The answer is seldom clear and usually depends upon the assumptions made and the time perspective taken. If it is assumed that these nursing hours will be allocated to other patients, and fewer nurses will be needed, then the costs definitely are variable. But if the "saved" hours are absorbed in the same amount of patient care or more personal time, then it is not clear whether nursing time should be considered fixed or variable. Economists tend to designate these hours variable because in the long run either fewer nurses will be required or increased productivity should result; but administrators of hospitals think of nursing costs as being fixed in the short run. The reader, therefore, must decide what makes the most sense under the particular circumstances at hand. From a policy- or decision-maker's standpoint, it is critical that costs be examined carefully to estimate which costs are truly variable to the program or institution that is affected by the medication under study.

Fixed and Variable Costs

This study compared the cost-effectiveness of 17 different antibiotic regimens for three clinical conditions. The costs of personnel and supplies were divided into fixed costs per regimen and variable costs per dose. (Weinstein et al. 1986)

Less obvious but important to many comprehensive economic evaluations are *indirect costs*. Indirect costs reflect the value of changes in health status and productivity that result from the health care intervention. These costs are termed "indirect" because they are not directly expended in the production of health care services or products and because they do not reflect the opportunity costs of the resources used in the process being evaluated. Some analysts prefer to classify these effects as negative benefits or negative consequences rather than as costs (recall the discussion of cost-benefit ratios in Chapter 3). The changes in health status may be valued in monetary or nonmonetary terms. In a CBA, all indirect costs are expressed in monetary terms. In a CUA and CEA, indirect costs may be measured in nonmonetary terms: however, losses in economic productivity may be incorporated into this the cost side of the equation as well.

Indirect Costs:

The monetary value of the changes in productivity that a patient experiences as a result of morbidity or mortality.

There are two main approaches to estimating the monetary value of indirect cost: the human capital approach, and the willingness to pay method. In the *human capital approach* to measuring indirect costs, changes in productivity are measured as the average earnings of persons in the labor force that will be lost or gained as a result of using a drug. The human capital approach does not attempt to value life per se, although it is sometimes interpreted in this way. Rather, it provides an estimate of the value of economic productivity changes that result from intervening in the course of the illness.

The Human Capital Approach

The cost of illness for diabetes was estimated including both direct and indirect costs. Indirect costs of the illness were measured for three separate conditions: short-term illnesses, permanent disability and death. Costs were estimated on the basis of the average labor market wage for men and women. (Jonsson 1983)

The human capital approach to valuing indirect costs is criticized on several counts. First, it ignores the psychosocial costs of illness, disability, and death, such as the disability associated with pain and suffering. There is no analytical reason, however, why the concepts of pain and suffering cannot be accounted for separately in such an analysis either as "costs" or "negative benefits". A second criticism is that the human capital approach implicitly undervalues any groups with lower paying jobs or individuals who are not employed, which would include the elderly, certain minority groups, and many females.

Economists have also devised ways to value the productivity of individuals who are not in the labor force. The *market value approach* measures an individual's contribution according to what monetary value that labor would fetch in the market place. For example, a homemaker's labor might be valued at the rate of house-cleaning services. (Of course, this severely undervalues the work of homemakers because they engage in much more activity than simply cleaning a house). An alternative method is the *opportunity cost approach* which values an individual's economic contribution according to the earnings that individual forgoes in order to remain in the home. This approach will usually result in larger estimated indirect costs.

Alternative Methods of Valuing Indirect Costs

This study examined the total economic costs associated with several major causes of death in the United States: cancer, heart disease, stroke, and motor vehicle accidents. The following table compares the results of using the market value approach and the opportunity cost approach.

	Total Costs (in billions)	
Condition	Market value	Opportunity cost
Cancer	$23.1	$27.6
Coronary heart disease	$13.7	$16.3
Stroke	$ 6.5	$ 8.1
Motor vehicle accidents	$14.4	$15.4

(Hartunian et al. 1980)

A second way of placing in monetary value on health and life is the *willingness to pay* methodology. There are several methods for obtaining a monetary value in this approach. One method entails explicitly asking individuals how much money they would be willing to spend to reduce the probability of illness or death. This method is limited by respondents' competence at assessing probabilities and by the validity of hypothetical judgments. Another method is to impute the value people place on their lives by observing certain behaviors. For example, people who work in high-risk occupations such as putting out oil rig fires ostensibly receive monetary compensation for their risk-tasking behavior. This method suffers from one major limitation. It is not necessary that people working in high-risk occupations receive additional monetary compensation for their risk-tasking; rather, they may simply be less risk-averse than the average person or they may receive utility other than cash for their efforts.

The willingness-to-pay method is preferred conceptually by economists because it theoretically takes into account a broader array of costs than does the human capital approach. Depending on how the data are obtained, the willingness-to-pay method may include lost wages (the costs that the human capital approach measures) as well as intangible effects that include pain, suffering, and other psychosocial costs. A drawback of the willingness-to-pay methodology is that the estimates will vary based on the initial wealth of the individual. For example, wealthy people are probably *willing* to pay more to avoid risks than are less wealthy people simply because they are *able* to pay more.

Another technique in measuring and valuing otherwise intangible costs is *utility analysis*. Utility analysis is covered in detail in Chapter 6, "Assessing Consequences" and in Chapter 12; however, it should be remembered that utility analysis can be used to measure costs that might otherwise be considered intangible.

5.3 Determinants of the Types of Costs To Incorporate into Analysis

Three major considerations dictate the type of resource change that is valued in monetary terms in a socioeconomic evaluation. These include: a) the type of analysis to be performed, e.g., CBA, CEA, or CUA; b) the perspective taken in the study; and c) the alternatives with which the technology in question will be compared.

5.3.1 Type of Analysis

The first determinant of costs to include in an evaluation is the type of analysis that will be performed. In CBA, all costs and all benefits are presented in monetary terms; therefore, all components of the equation are estimated as monetary costs. This entails placing monetary values on outcomes not normally represented in economic terms, such as a life saved. As has been noted previously, a CBA might include only those consequences that are easily expressed in monetary values, such as changes in productivity, but might ignore changes in health status or quality of life. In such a case, a narrower range of consequences would be incorporated posing a potentially major limitation. In CEA and CUA all direct costs and sometimes indirect costs (e.g., productivity) are valued in dollar terms, however, health outcomes are not expressed monetarily.

5.3.2 Alternatives

A second major determinant of the types of costs to incorporate into an economic analysis is the *alternative* with which the technology will be compared. Counts of resources for alternative scenarios should be comparable. For example, from a societal perspective, a comparison of home health care and institutional health care for chronically ill patients should include the variable costs for heating, electricity, food, and rent in the home care setting because these items will be incorporated into the total costs for the institution[1]. Of course, from the perspective of a third party payer, some of these costs may not be germane.

5.3.3 Perspective

From each viewpoint there are differing information needs and criteria of evaluation. Perspective is important because what is cost-effective for one party (for

---

[1] These costs should be included only if they are truly variable, that is, if they would change once the individual no longer lived in the home.

example, the hospital) may not be cost-effective for another (for example, a third party payer). Thus, specific costs may or may not be appropriate from different perspectives. Table 5.1 summarizes the types of cost that would be examined from each perspective. Although studies are performed from every perspective, the policy- or decision-maker should be aware that only the societal perspective considers all costs relevant to society as a whole. Any other perspective may result in decisions that may be nonoptimal.

Table 5.1. How perspective determines costs

Perspective	Costs of primary interest
Societal	All medical and nonmedical costs: Hospitalization Long-term care Home care Social welfare services Productivity losses (indirect costs) Intangible costs
Third party payer	Charges that pertain to reimbursement of providers Average, not marginal cost
Health care provider	Variable costs that influence the expenses of providing health care
Patient	Costs that affect out-of-pocket payments Lost wages (indirect costs)
Employer	All insurable direct costs Lost wages (indirect costs)

5.4 Process of Identifying Costs

When identifying costs, researchers begin by enumerating the resources that are required to produce a certain outcome. For example, this may entail counting the number of tests, doctors' visits, and number of days in the hospital. A description of the pathways of clinical management can be most helpful in this process. These pathways specify the inputs that are required to produce certain outcomes. This requires an accounting of the resources consumed (labor, equipment, and supplies), the manner in which they are combined, and the outcomes or changes in health status that are produced. As can be imagined, this can become a very complex process.

At this point, monetary values are not explicitly considered, rather, the focus is on the inputs and the outputs in terms of resource use. The process of resource identification can be fairly crude or it may be painstakingly detailed. Generally, if the socioeconomic differences between the alternatives are large, the types of resources enumerated and the method of identifying them may be less precise than when smaller differences are expected.

Identifying Resources: Method 1

In an analysis of the cost-effectiveness of a cholesterol-lowering medication, the impact of the drug was simulated by using epidemiological data. Gross costs were estimated for the intervention and cardiovascular disease events such as angina pectoris and myocardial infarction; however, no detailed empirical data were gathered. Although there may be considerable error associated with these methods, the study provides an approximation of expenditures. (Oster and Epstein 1987)

Identifying Resources: Method 2

At the other extreme is a detailed cost-accounting exercise to detect very small differences in production costs of a commonly administered intravenous antibiotic. This analysis used the principles of industrial engineering, component enumeration, and time-motion studies to compare the actual production costs of three different antibiotics. The costs of acquiring, preparing, and administering the drugs were broken into discrete work steps. These were analyzed to determine which steps varied across the drugs. Personnel time, supplies, and equipment were thoroughly measured within each step to describe the resources required to provide antibiotic therapy. (Eisenberg et al. 1984).

5.5 Assigning Monetary Values to Resources

Estimating the monetary value of resources is another area in which analysts must often compromise between the ideal and the pragmatic. It can be a time-consuming and expensive process to identify accurately the true economic cost of a medication. This would entail describing all costs involved in production, marketing, distribution, storage, and prescribing to patients. Overheads allocated to that medication must be estimated. Marginal as opposed to average costs must be computed. Because this process can be laborious, compromises are justifiable. Analysts must weight the value of the information: will the estimates that result from this process of counting the most minute cost element be considerably more accurate than simply using charges? Given the necessity of providing information at a reasonable cost, the use of charges as a proxy for costs is justifiable as long as there is no indication that the two are widely divergent.

As noted in Chap. 2, in a truly competitive market, prices of goods and services would represent their marginal opportunity costs. However, cross-subsidization, cost-shifting, and other forces in the medical care market have resulted in a wide discrepancy between marginal production costs and prices or charges. For example, there are several sources of cost distortion in Europe. First, prices of medications tend to be fixed within each European country and these prices may or may not reflect costs. Second, there tends to be no specific charge system for resources used within the hospital sector. Rather, there is only an overall daily rate for hospital services. Third, there tends to be no cost-reporting: thus, it may be difficult accurately to determine the price of individual resources utilized.

Nevertheless, the use of charges as a proxy for economic costs can represent a reasonable compromise under certain conditions and given appropriate precautions. Here again, the perspective of the analysis should be a major determinant of the valuation procedure. From the perspective of a third party payer, sickness fund, or patient, charges are the cost of interest while opportunity costs are irrelevant. From the hospital's perspective, its own expenditures are moor important. From the ideal social perspective, the actual costs of production are the most relevant costs to include in the analysis. Use of charges is also a reasonable compromise when comparative, as opposed to absolute, costing is required. For example, suppose two groups of patients receiving different treatments are being compared with one another. If there is no reason to believe that the cost-to-charge ratios across categories of services are different, then charges can be acceptable depictions of the magnitude of differences between the two groups. Nonetheless, comparable cost-to-charge ratios must be empirically demonstrated and not assumed and if bias is suspected its direction and likely size ought to be discussed.

5.6 Monetary Valuation of Consequences

When outcomes or consequences can be expressed in monetary values, these values are sometimes substracted from the cost side of the equation. Savings in health care resources are then considered to be "negative costs".

Positive and Negative Costs

In a study of the use of estrogen among postmenopausal women, the following cost-effectiveness equation was examined:

$$\frac{C}{E}=\frac{\Delta C_{Rx}+\Delta C_{SE}-\Delta C_{Morb}}{\Delta Y-\Delta Y_{SE}-\Delta Y_{Morb}+\Delta Y_{Symp}}$$

Where: C_{Rx} = costs of treatment
C_{SE} = costs caused by side effects of treatment
C_{Morb} = savings associated with preventing other conditions such as hip fracture

Note that even though C_{Morb} represents a benefit of the treatment it appears on the cost side of the equation because it has a monetary value. (Weinstein 1980)

Recall from Chap. 3 that, when reporting cost-benefit ratios, the ratio will differ according to whether the savings are subtracted from the numerator or added to the denominator.

5.7 Specific Types of Costs

Table 5.2 lists direct and indirect costs that may be appropriate to examine during a socioeconomic evaluation. Not all costs will be included in every study, rather, this listing should serve to sensitize the reader to the conventional categories of costs and specific examples within each category.

Table 5.2. Types of costs

Directs costs

Direct medical costs

- Institutional inpatient care
- Institutional outpatient services
- Home health care
- Physician services
- Ancillary services
- Volunteers
- Overhead allocated to the technology
  - Fixed costs of utilities
  - Space
  - Storage
  - Support services: laundry, housekeeping, administration
- Variable costs of utilities
- Medications: prescription and nonprescription
  - Drug costs
  - Treating side effects or toxicity of medications
  - Prophylaxis of side effects
  - Ordering and inventorying
  - Preparation
  - Training in new procedures
  - Dispensing and administration
  - Monitoring
- Devices and appliances
- Drugs, supplies, devices provided by household
- Research and development
- Diagnostic tests
- Treatment services
- Prevention services
- Rehabilitation
- Training and education

Direct nonmedical costs

- Care provided by family and friends
- Transportation to and from medical services
- Child care
- Housekeeping
- Modification of home to accommodate patients
- Social services
- Program Evaluation

Indirect costs (May also be treated as negative consequences)

- Time and productivity
  - Change in productivity resulting from change in health status
    - Morbidity
    - Mortality
    - Averted illness
  - Lost productivity while on job
    - Absenteeism
  - Income lost by family members
  - Forgone leisure time
  - Time spent by patient seeking medical services
  - Time spent by family and friends attending patient (e.g., hospital visitations)

Intangible costs

- Psychosocial costs
  - Apprehension; anxiety
  - Grief and loss of well-being associated with:
    - Impending death
    - Disfigurement
    - Disability
    - Economic and physical dependence
    - Loss of job
    - Loss of opportunity for promotion and education
  - Social isolation
  - Family conflict
- Valuations others put on patient's health and well-being
- Pain
- Changes in social functioning and activities of daily living

5.8 Common Problems in Estimating Costs

In reading socioeconomic evaluations, the reader will encounter a number of problems that arise repeatedly in estimating costs. Table 5.3 summarizes some of the more common dilemmas faced by researchers, along with acceptable compromises for solving these dilemmas.

Table 5.3. The ideal and the pragmatic in estimating costs

Ideal standard	Pragmatic response
Enumerate all resources involved in producing the service or technology under scrutiny	Weigh the amount of information expected from all categories of costs; include easily measurable costs and those costs that are expected to differ considerably between patients
	Make explicit in the report which costs are not included and how this omission is expected to affect the analysis. Consult clients
Use marginal rather than average costs	If marginal costs do not vary a great deal, or if capital costs are not large, use of average costs may be acceptable
Use opportunity costs rather than market price (charges)	Charges may be acceptable when the cost-to-charge ratios across service categories (e.g., hospital departments) are similar or when utilization across charge categories is similar across patients
	Charges may be used when comparative as opposed to absolute costing is required
	From certain perspectives (e.g., the third party payer), charges are the value of interest. Assess any likely bias
Include indirect costs	Include when it is expected that productivity will be lost or gained
	If large differences are expected in direct costs, it may not be necessary to include indirect costs if they are expected to vary in the same direction
Indirect costs should include lost market productivity as well as personal costs such as forgone leisure time, time spent by family and friends	Use market wage rate for patient, recognizing that this is an underestimate of true indirect costs (human capital approach)
	Estimate indirect costs using the willingness to pay method and attempt to elicit or approximate a broader range of costs than market productivity. Consider client's perspective
Include overheads	Omitting overheads is justifiable if the technology is marginal to the overall enterprise, that is, overhead costs would remain unchanged is the technology were eliminated

Table 5.3. (continued)

Ideal standard	Pragmatic response
Account for future efficiences that result from learning or technological development	Estimate costs under average working conditions using sensitivity analysis[a]
Account for the inefficiencies of average operating conditions as opposed to ideal study conditions	Estimate costs under average working conditions using sensitivity analysis[a]
Account for the inefficiencies of highly skilled clinicians performing tasks that less skilled personnel can perform	Estimate costs under average working conditions using sensitivity analysis[a]
For rapidly changing technologies perform evaluations repeatedly rather than at only one point in time	Estimate costs under average working conditions using sensitivity analysis[a]
Include resources that are "free" from the perspective of the provider	From a societal perspective, "free" costs (e.g., patient time and volunteer time) should be included. Use market wage rates. For resources that are already owned by provider, estimate alternative use value
Do not include transfer payments	Even though transfer payments (such as taxes and disability payments) are not economic costs, they may be pertinent in a study from an agent's budgetary perspective. Keep distinct from cost analysis

[a] Sensitivity analysis is a process in which different values of critical variables are used for the analysis in order to assess the impact of changing these values. It is described in detail in Chap. 7.

5.9 Conclusion

The estimation of costs is limited by researchers' knowledge base regarding how to assess direct and indirect costs as well as limitations in their ability to assign monetary values to resources. Ideally, the analyst should attempt to include all of the costs identified in Table 5.2; however, practical compromises must be made. Some forms of costs may be disregarded because they are known, *a priori,* to be virtually identical for the services or technologies being compared. Other costs may be so small that their numerical impact on the analysis is likely to be negligible, and thus collecting these data would not be worthwhile. In general, the evaluation should focus on forms of cost that are expected to diverge significantly from one another. Costs that are not normally considered, such as direct nonmedical expenses and indirect costs, should be included when a major effect of the drug may be reflected in these categories. In the case of studies conducted for specified clients, exclusions and compromises should be discussed with clients at both the study design stage and as the study progresses. Assumptions made by analysts that turn out to be unacceptable to clients may vitiate an otherwise good study and relegate it to gathering dust on a library shelf.

6 Assessing Consequences

6.1 Introduction

The consequences of using a medication reflect both the drug's immediate effectiveness and the subsequent results of using the medication, such as adverse reactions, the need for further diagnostic evaluations, and the need for additional therapy. A medication's impact may be favorable or unfavorable. It will be favorable insofar as the treatment is successful and treatment costs decrease. On the other hand, the impact will be unfavorable when a medication is ineffective, has adverse side effects, and treatment costs increase. Some of the effects of a medication may be indeterminate. There may be considerable uncertainty about the precise nature, magnitude, or even the direction of the consequences. Some consequences cannot be anticipated by the researcher and thus remain unmeasured in the study; however, there may be important outcomes that could change conclusions about the use of the medication. The previous chapter addressed some economic consequences during the description of the evaluation of costs. This chapter elaborates by focusing on the evaluation of the health consequences of a medication.

6.2 Types of Consequences

There are three general categories of consequences: clinical, psychosocial, and economic. These are summarized in Table 6.1.

6.2.1 Clinical Consequences

The clinical impact of a medication is the fundamental outcome of interest. Indeed, without a positive and substantial clinical effect, a medication should not be approved for use and would not require socioeconomic evaluation. Clinical consequences are derived from the world of medicine and include measures of morbidity and mortality.

Changes in *mortality* are measured as the number of lives saved or the years of life saved as a result of using the medication; however, medical interventions seldom result in a simple life or death outcome. There are inevitably survivors who are in less than perfect health as a result of the disease under study. Nonetheless, many socioeconomic studies report only crude outcome measures such as mortality, which may not be adequate for the policy issues at hand.

Table 6.1. Types of consequences

Clinical consequences
Morbidity
Cure of acute conditions
Control of chronic conditions
Reduction of disability
Mortality
Lives saved
Years of life saved
Other (intermediate outcomes)
Cases found
Correct diagnoses
Use of health care resources
Cases prevented
Changes in behavior
Psychosocial consequences
Intangibles
Quality of life
Utility
Quality-adjusted life years
Economic consequences
Use of health resources, monetary or nonmonetary
Hospital days
Physician visits
Other medications or services
Nonmonetary economic effects
Absenteeism
Job changes
Productivity

Effectiveness Measured as Changes in Mortality
Example 1

Three forms of treatment for esophageal varices were compared in a Japanese study: sclerotherapy (injecting a substance into the varicose veins in the esophagus to scar them shut), surgical interruption of the veins, and surgical shunting of the veins. Effectiveness of the treatments was compared by examining the survival rates for each treatment. The results were expressed in terms of yen/survivor. (Sasaki and Eisenberg 1987)

Example 2

In a study of the economic impact of swine-flu vaccination, the noneconomic benefits associated with the vaccination program were measured as the "number of years of life that would be lost if an epidemic occurred". (Schoenbaum et al. 1976a)

Changes in *morbidity* include the cure of acute conditions, such as a successfully treated infection, and the control of chronic conditions, such as maintaining blood pressure within a normal range, preventing diabetic ketoacidosis, or reducing psychiatric symptoms. Again, these traditional clinical measures of effectiveness do not take into account the quality of life, but changes in health status are clearly evaluated. Clinical measures also do not consider the socioeconomic consequences of improvements in health status.

Effectiveness Measured as Changes in Morbidity

> This study compared the cost-effectiveness of broad-spectrum antibiotics using these measures of effectiveness:
> 1. Number of patients clinically cured
> 2. Number of bacterial strains eradicated according to bacteriological tests
> 3. Number of patients with adverse reactions. (Norrby et al. 1986)

The primary limitation of using only medical measures of effectiveness in an analysis is that, unless the clinical outcomes are expressed in similar units, it is difficult to compare results analytically. To address this limitation, other measures such as economic values, utility, and quality of life have been used to compare treatments with different outcomes.

Other clinical measures that might be used in socioeconomic evaluations include changes in *health care resource utilization* such as reducing days spent in bed and reducing institutionalization. These measures are usually expressed in monetary values.

6.2.2 Psychosocial Consequences

Psychosocial consequences have often been relegated to a category called "intangible" effects, namely, they were not considered measurable or quantifiable. With advances in measurement, many of these previously intangible effects are now being examined in socioeconomic evaluations. These advances in measurement have occurred in the areas of quality of life and the assessment of utility values.

Outcomes of Antihypertensive Therapy

> Clinical measures of blood pressure are the most common means of assessing the effectiveness of antihypertensive medications. This study compared three medications that were roughly equivalent in clinical effectiveness but that had very different implications for quality of life. Quality of life was measured as general well-being, physical symptoms, and sexual dysfunction among other factors. (Croog et al. 1986)

Psychosocial consequences include changes in pain, anxiety, self-esteem, and ability to perform expected social roles. Two methods used to quantify psychosocial effects include quality of life assessment and the assignment of utility values. The concept of quality of life was discussed in Chap. 3 and is described in greater detail in Chap. 10.

Utility analysis consists of measuring health outcomes in some common, nonmonetary unit in order to compare different types of outcomes. The reason that this is necessary is best illustrated by an example. Consider a comparison of two medications used to treat hypertension. Both are equally effective in reducing blood pressure; thus, estimates of years of life saved for the two drugs would be comparable. However, each drug has a different adverse reaction: lethargy and decreased cognitive function for one, and impotence for the other. How can these two drugs be evaluated? How can we value the health state produced by one drug compared with the health state resulting from the other? One way to compare the medications would to be perform utility analysis, which directly elicits patients' preferences of one health state compared with another.

Utility Analysis:

A method of measuring health outcomes in terms of the preferences that individuals express for being in that health state. Provides a common unit with which to compare interventions with widely divergent outcomes.

One common method of obtaining "utility values" involves asking people (medical professionals, patients, or healthy people) to assign values to various states of health. The responses from numerous people are combined and the resulting utility values are assigned to the health states associated with a treatment or condition. There are several means of obtaining and using utility values. These are described in detail in Chap. 12.

Utility Values for Health States

When utility values are estimated for health states, perfect health is generally assigned a value of 1.0 and death is assigned a value of zero. The following table presents the utility values for certain health states as presented in one study.

Health state	Utility value
Healthy	1.00 (reference)
Life with menopausal symptoms	0.99
Mild angina	0.90
Kidney transplant	0.84
Some physical limitation with occasional pain	0.67
Being deaf, dumb, or blind	0.39
Dead	0.00 (reference)
Confined to bed with severe pain	<0.00

These values were obtained by asking various groups of people to rate these states of health. Some groups consisted of members of the general public; some were experts, some were patients. (Torrance 1987)

6.2.3 Economic Consequences

Economic consequences may be expressed in financial or in qualitative terms. Essentially, when monetary values are assigned to the effects of a medication, the health and psychosocial consequences of a medication are being expressed in financial terms. Rather than simply counting the lives saved or the days of disability that are averted, monetary values are ascribed to health resource outcomes. In this vein, health consequences might be expressed in terms of the cost of avoided days of hospitalization. Alternatively, some economic consequences may not be easily quantifiable and are expressed in their natural units. For example, one economic outcome of a successful treatment may be reduced worker absenteeism.

Economic Consequences Expressed in Nonmonetary Terms

This study examined the cost-benefit of alternative treatment regimens for mental illness. Among the benefits included were:
1. Number of days employed per year
2. Percentage of days missed from job
3. Number of beneficial job changes
4. Number of detrimental job changes
5. Percentage of patients who had a savings account

Note that these consequences all have economic implications; however, these factors are not readily translated into monetary values. What is important is that the consequences were not ignored just because no monetary values could be assigned to them. (Weisbrod et al. 1980)

Alternatively, life itself might be expressed in monetary terms. There are several methods of valuing life. The *human capital* and *willingness to pay* methods are described in Chapter 5 under indirect costs.

Economic Consequences Expressed in Monetary Terms

In a study of prenatal screening and immunization against hepatitis B, one major economic consequence was examined: lost productivity that resulted from chronic liver disease or death that was a sequel of hepatitis B. Lost productivity was measured as the potential lifetime earnings that were lost. (Arevalo and Washington 1988)

6.3 Determinants of Which Consequences Are Included in an Analysis

Ideally a socioeconomic evaluation should examine all possible consequences; however, practical considerations limit the extent to which we can examine outcomes of therapy. There are three main determinants of how consequences are conceptualized, measured, and valued:
1. the type of study,
2. the research question addressed in the study, and
3. the perspective of the study.

6.3.1 Type of Study

Recall from Chap. 3 that when input costs are measured in a socioeconomic evaluation they are always measured as monetary values. It is in the measurement and valuation of consequences that the types of socioeconomic evaluations differ.

While CEA measures health outcomes in natural units, CBA values health consequences in monetary terms. The advantage of valuing health outcomes monetarily is that widely divergent outcomes can be compared. The disadvantage is that outcomes such as years of life saved must be expressed in economic terms, which is a difficult, controversial, and imperfect process. As CUA gains more prominence and its techniques are refined by researchers, it will become a particularly useful compromise because it attempts to capture the gestalt of the total health and economic consequences in units that are comparable across a wide variety of outcomes.

6.3.2 Research Question

The research question asks, in part, what is the range of possible health outcomes from using the medication? These outcomes are described when the pathways of clinical management for the medication are specified (see Chap. 4).

Different medications produce different effects; thus, different consequences will be examined. An antihypertensive medication should be evaluated for outcomes such as adverse reactions, reduced blood pressure, and reduced cardiovascular and cerebrovascular complications. A vaccine should be evaluated for cases of disease prevented and complications from the vaccination. In both cases, economic consequences can be evaluated as well.

The Research Question as a Determinant of Which Consequences Are Assessed

The objective of this study was to assess the quality of life effects of three antihypertensive medications: propranolol, captopril, and methyldopa. Even though it is likely that the medications differed in their efficacy in reducing blood pressure and, thus, in their associated years of life saved, these outcomes were not assessed, nor were economic outcomes assessed. The outcomes of interest were adverse reactions from the drugs such as lethargy, sexual disorders, headaches, dizziness, and nausea. (Croog et al. 1986)

6.3.3 Perspective

The perspective of the study is also important in determining what types of consequences are analyzed in a study. As described in Chap. 4, all consequences, no matter how far flung, potentially can be included in a study performed from the societal perspective. Not only would immediate effects on patients' physical, social, and personal lives be examined, but long-term consequences would be assessed as well. The societal perspective might include analyses of broader social consequences such as changes in resource allocation and changes in economic productivity. From the narrow fiscal viewpoint of the third party payer, however, only those consequences that are relevant to reimbursement of medical services need to be included in the analysis. There will be less concern with consequences that are personal to the patient such as lost productivity, relatively small changes in quality of life (such as improved convenience), and patient time.

From the perspective of the patient who is insured and is not totally responsible for paying the medical bill, financial consequences are not so relevant, although quality of life is extremely pertinent. From the physician's perspective, the primary consequences are health outcomes. Indeed, physicians and the medical profession as a whole have been criticized for not emphasizing quality of life assessment. All nonsocietal perspectives tend to be suboptimal and thus lead to substantial distortions in the interpretation of the true value of a technology.

6.4 Medication Compliance

Noncompliance with therapeutic regimes is a major problem in clinical medicine. Estimates of noncompliance range between 10% and 90%, depending on the regimen, the drug, patient characteristics, and characteristics of the treatment setting (Sackett and Snow 1979). As a result, perfect adherence to therapy should not be assumed during socioeconomic evaluations of drugs. In clinical trials of medications, researchers generally go to great lengths to ensure that patients in the study are indeed taking their prescribed medication; however, this is not always possible in the routine clinical setting. Patients may take their medications erratically or cease altogether, they may fail to attend clinic at the recommended intervals for observation, or they may fail to obtain necessary laboratory tests to check on potential adverse reactions to the drug.

Compliance:

The extent to which patients' health-related behaviors conform to the recommendations made by clinicians; also termed adherence.

The primary effect of noncompliance is to reduce potential benefits of treatment and to exacerbate disease. Erratic medication-taking reduces the effectiveness of the drug and may lead to complete cessation. Thus, the health consequences of a medication may be considerably attenuated as a result of noncompliance. If noncompliance is expected to be a significant problem, then it should be included in the anylsis.

Accounting for Noncompliance in Socioeconomic Evaluations

This study examined the cost-effectiveness of several different treatment regimens for tuberculosis. One of the major differences between the treatments was the length of therapy required. Based on the assumption that compliance is a function of time, it was estimated that 21% of patients will discontinue therapy after 6 months, 38% will be noncompliant at 12 months, and 51% will be noncompliant at 18 months. The effectiveness of each regimen was examined in light of these noncompliance rates. (Barnum 1986)

6.5 Conclusion

This chapter has described the "other half" of socioeconomic evaluations: the consequences of using the medication. These consequences are divided into three general categories: a) health consequences, b) psychosocial consequences, and c) economic consequences.

Measuring consequences is a challenging task for the researcher. Many important outcomes are not quantifiable in monetary terms with even a modicum of confidence; thus CBA is not always feasible. Clinical consequences such as morbidity and mortality can be useful; however, these measures often do not capture the full range of outcomes that result from treatment. Quality of life assessment and utility analysis are means of measuring those effects that have previously been considered intangible or nonquantifiable.

Table 6.2. The ideal and the pragmatic in assessing consequences

Ideal standard	Pragmatic response
Measure all health consequences of the technology	Measure only mortality when the differences between the alternatives are expected to be great and the measurement of other consequences will only confirm these results
	When only a limited range of outcomes are examined, state in the report which outcomes are missing and how their inclusion might affect the results
	Measure intermediate outcomes (e.g., cases found) when ultimate outcomes are distant. Extrapolate the health impact and clinical significance of these intermediate outcomes
	The range of relevant consequences in studies conducted from a non-societal perspective may be more restricted. Consult potential client
Assess "intangible" consequences	Use utility analysis or quality of life assessment. Acknowledge what intangible consequences are not captured in these measures. Consult clients about this
	Array the intangible effects of a technology, making the reader aware of their existence but do not incorporate them in the analysis
Measure consequences as accurately as possible	Use sensitivity analysis[a] for outcomes that are measured with considerable uncertainty
For a CEA measure all outcomes in the same units	If the outcomes of a technology cannot be expressed in the same units, array the outcomes in their natural units and report results for all measures of effectiveness, e.g., lives saved, days of morbidity, days of disability could all be reported as outcomes of one intervention
For a CBA, value all consequences in dollar terms	See Chap. 5 for a discussion of the difficulties inherent in assigning monetary values

[a] Sensitivity analysis is a process in which different values of critical variables are used for the analysis in order to assess the impact of changing these values. It is described in detail in Chap. 7.

Although the goal of socioeconomic evaluation is to assess the full range of consequences that result from the use of a medication, this is often not feasible. Researchers must be prepared to compromise. Table 6.2 examines the ideal standards which guide evaluators and the accepted compromises that they often are compelled to make.

In general, researchers should begin by enumerating the full range of consequences that are expected based on the clinical evidence that is available. They should evaluate which consequences are most relevant and which are most likely to differ among the alternatives compared. They should examine consequences to appraise which are measurable in monetary terms, which are measurable in natural units, and which can be valued using quality of life or utility measures. Finally, in reporting results, researchers should make explicit which outcomes are *not* included in the final results and what the impact of these omissions might be on the interpretation of results. Often it is helpful to provide a qualitative description of those forms of consequences that are not included in the quantitative analysis and, as always, if the study is being conducted for a specified client, the client's views about omissions should be thoroughly investigated and fully represented in the analysis.

7 Adjusting Costs and Consequences

7.1 Introduction

The numbers reported in socioeconomic evaluations usually need to be adjusted by researchers for at least one of two reasons: either the costs and/or consequences are incurred or accrue over time; or there is considerable uncertainty regarding their true value. This adjustment of costs and consequences allows a more accurate description of the socioeconomic impact of a medication. These two adjustments are termed *discounting* and *sensitivity analysis*.

7.2 Discounting

When costs or consequences occur in the future, or when costs and consequences do not occur at the same time, the values should be adjusted by discounting. The principle behind discounting is the *positive value of time preference*, which results in a social as well as a private preference for postponing costs and obtaining benefits as soon as possible. In other words, people generally prefer to have their benefits sooner and their costs later. This means that benefits in the present have greater value than benefits in the future[1] and costs in the present are more serious than costs in the future because money available now can be invested to yield higher future returns.

Discounting:

> The process whereby future costs or benefits are mathematically reduced to their present value.

The process of discounting involves reducing events in the future (either costs or consequences) by an appropriate factor called the discount rate. Discounting is performed by weighting future events by the discount factor in order to reduce all future values to present values. Mathematically, it can be thought of as the reverse

[1] The reader should note that discounting is not an adjustment for inflation. This discussion of discounting may raise questions regarding the impact of inflation on costs and consequences that occur far in the future. In general, analysts deal with inflation by converting all monetary values into constant prices, usually, today's prices.

of computing a return on investment. In order to compute the present discounted value of a stream of costs incurred on a yearly basis throughout the lifetime of the technology, the following equation is used:

$$C_{\mathrm{pdv}} = C_0 + \frac{C_1}{(1+r)} + \frac{C_2}{(1+r)^2} + \cdots + \frac{C_{\mathrm{n}}}{(1+r)^n}$$

where:
C_{pdv} = present discounted value of costs
C_0 = immediate costs
C_1 = costs in year 1
C_2 = costs in year 2
n = last year technology is used
r = discount rate
$1/(1+r)$ = discount factor

Although there is consensus that discounting should be conducted in socioeconomic evaluations, there is less agreement on exactly what the discount rate should be. That rate chosen is important, however, especially for a medication that has predicted cost savings or benefits that occur well into the future and for alternatives having different patterns of cost and consequence over time. The higher the discount rate, the less value is placed on costs or consequences that are incurred farther in the future. Thus, for preventive therapies whose costs are immediate while the benefits are not expected to accrue for many years, a high discount rate would diminish the net benefits of the program, while a low discount rate would make the net benefits appear larger. In general the use of discount rates should be subject to sensitivity analysis (see below).

When using a discount rate of 5%, a $100 cost that is incurred 20 years into the future has a discounted present value of $37.69. Postponing these costs for 50 years reduces them to a present value of $8.72. The original $100 has been considerably diminished during the process of discounting; thjus discuonted costs that occur far in the future often have little impact on the calculations in a socioeconomic evaluation.

In the socioeconomic evaluation literature, a 3% to 5% rate is commonly used for the base estimate, or best guess. It is also common to look at the effect of using other estimates of the discount rate that may range from 0% to 10%. Some countries specify which discount rate should be used for projects in the public sector or using public expenditure.

Two guidelines can be used to determine whether discounting should be performed in a particular study. If all costs and consequences occur within a short period, say one year, then discounting is not necessary. However, when costs and consequences occur in the future or, if they occur at different times, then discounting should be used.

Although it may appear logical to discount costs, the thought of discounting noneconomic values such as a year of life saved may be troublesome to some readers. Failure to discount consequences, however, can lead to illogical conclusions. If future costs are discounted but future consequences are not, then it would be possible to conclude that health programs should be postponed indefinitely because they will have lower future costs for benefits that are equivalent to those experienced today.

A topic that illustrates the relevance of discounting is the distinction between prevalence-based and incidence-based socioeconomic evaluations. *Prevalence* is an epidemiological term that refers to the current number of persons afflicted with a certain condition at one point in time. *Incidence* refers to the number of new cases of the disease that arises over a specified period. Another way of looking at incidence is to consider it the probability of a healthy person developing the condition during, say, a one-year period. Because chronic diseases last a long time, they tend to have a high prevalence rate, even if their incidence is fairly low. Acute diseases, such as the common cold, have a short duration, high incidence, and relative to their incidence, a low prevalence.

A *prevalence-based socioeconomic evaluation* ascribes the costs of the condition to the year in which the condition actually occurs. For example, the costs and consequences of treating a stroke that results from untreated hypertension might be attributed to the year in which the stroke occurs. Typically, a prevalence-based analysis will estimate the burden of stroke to a nation in a certain year.

A Prevalence-Based Study

This report examined the costs of illness of smoking by estimating the costs of four major conditions associated with smoking: cancer, diseases of the circulatory system, diseases of the respiratory system, and injuries caused by fires. The authors estimated the total costs of each of these diseases and the proportion of each condition that was attributable to smoking. They reported the direct health care costs of treating smoking-related conditions that occurred in 1976, the lifetime earnings that were lost because of morbidity or mortality that occurred in 1976 and the property costs of smoking-related fires. Lifetime earnings were discounted at a 4% rate. The total economic impact of smoking (in 1976 dollars) was over $27 billion. Direct health costs alone amounted to over $8 billion. Because this study examined the costs of *current* smoking-related conditions, it is a prevalence-based study. (Luce and Schweitzer 1978)

On the other hand, an *incidence-based approach* considers the present value of the stream of costs and consequences of a disease associated with a cohort of individuals at risk for the disease. In the example of stroke, the costs of the disease would typically begin for an asymptomatic group in, say 1988, and extend through their lifetime. For chronic diseases of long duration, the cost figures that result from the incidence-based approach will be smaller than those obtained from the prevalence-based approach. This happens because the costs occur over a long period and future costs are discounted to their present value.

An Incidence-Based Study

This study examined the costs of three smoking-related illnesses: emphysema, lung cancer, and coronary heart disease. The authors started with a group of patients who were healthy, utilized epidemiological data regarding the probabilities of developing these conditions, and then estimated the costs of future morbidity and mortality associated with smoking. All costs were discounted at a 3% rate. The total economic costs of smoking ranged from $1046 for a woman who smoked less than one packer per day to $61 304 for a man who smoked more than two packs per day. (Oster et al. 1984)

The incidence-based approach is appropriate when examining preventive measures such as a vaccination program. This is because expenditures occur at one point in time, or over a period of time, while the benefits accrue in the future. The prevalence-based approach is best used when scrutinizing treatments that have more or less immediate effects.

7.3 Sensitivity Analysis

Often during socioeconomic evaluations precise data are unavailable for some variables. Under such conditions of uncertainty, analysts often make a "best estimate" based on the information available to them. If there is uncertainty regarding the values of particular variables, it is necessary to examine how different plausible values affect the results that are reached. This technique, termed sensitivity analysis, is used when analysts lack information as a way of testing the assumptions made in the analysis. Because of frequent limitations in data, sensitivity analysis is almost always useful.

Sensitivity Analysis:

An analytical process that examines the effect on the results of an analysis of changing the values of key variables.

When researchers lack information, costs and consequences cannot be estimated with certainly. This occurs when: a) production functions cannot be clearly traced, b) when the use of resources is uncertain, or c) when a distribution of data, rather than precise values, is available.

Under these conditions, several estimates of variables such as costs can be computed. Often, the results are expressed as a best estimate (or base case), a high estimate, and a low estimate. The two extreme values would represent a most conservative and least conservative estimate of the impact of the medication. Generally, it is good to select values for benefits that tend to err on the conservative side and vice versa for costs. Thus, if the research hypothesis is that a new drug is more cost-effective than an existing course of therapy, conservative estimates of uncertain benefits would tend to bias the results against the hypothesis. This makes the study more likely to be believable even to a skeptic.

Sensitivity analysis is useful not only for the analysis of monetary costs, but also for testing uncertainty associated with nonmonetary costs and consequences.

Sensitivity Analysis on Monetary and Nonmonetary Variables

This study examined the cost-effectiveness of pneumococcal vaccine. Precise data for several monetary and nonmonetary variables were unavailable; thus sensitivity analysis was performed. These uncertain variables were arrayed in a table, part of which is reproduced here:

Variables	*Values*		
	Base case	High value	Low value
Cost of vaccination	$11.37	–	$3.45
Duration of immunity	8 years	72 years	3 years
Efficacy rate	80%	100%	40%
Proportion of pneumonia that is pneumococcal	15%	35%	10%

Only one of these variables is a monetary cost. The other three variables are measures of the efficacy of the vaccine. Note that no high value is presented for cost of vaccination because only a base case and low value were known. (Willems et al. 1980)

Sensitivity analysis can help to point out critical values above or below which cost-effectiveness of a program cannot be shown. This is termed *threshold analysis*.

Threshold Analysis
Example 1

This study examined the cost-effectiveness of using a once daily antibiotic to treat osteomyelitis. Use of this antibiotic would enable patients to be treated at home. Using sensitivity analysis, the authors showed that if *none* of the patients who were discharged would be able to return to work immediately after hospitalization, then the new antibiotic would not be cost-effective. Cost-effectiveness would be greatest if *all* patients could return to work immediately. (Eisenberg and Kitz 1986)

Example 2

In another study, sensitivity analysis was performed to detect under what circumstances the cost-benefits associated with a vaccine would be eliminated: "The benefits of immunization are eliminated when the benefit-cost ratio is 1; this may happen when the rate of post-vaccination encephalitis reaches one case in 22,500 vaccinees, a rate almost eight-fold higher than the highest published rate ... We assumed that the cost of care of residual defects from post-vaccination encephalitis averages $5000 per year for 50 years ... The average cost would have to increase to $75,000 per year to reduce the cost-benefit ratio to 1." (Koplan et al. 1979)

Sensitivity analysis may also demonstrate that the conclusions reached under the base case assumption are vastly different from those reached under the high or low value. This would suggest that the overall analysis cannot be viewed as definitive.

Results That Are Sensitive to Assumptions

The cost-effectiveness of three different strategies for screening and immunization against hepatitis B was examined in this study. When assumptions regarding the estimated costs of treating hepatitis were varied, the results changed. For example, when it was assumed that treatment costs for the disease were only half the best estimate ($227/case), then the attack rate[2] for hepatitis B in the population would have to be 10% before immunization was cost-saving. On the other hand, if treatment costs were four times the best estimate ($1812/case), then the attack rate could be as small as 2%. (Mulley et al. 1982)

Alternatively, sensitivity analysis may show that the same conclusions are drawn regardless of which values are used in the analysis. This means that the analysis is insensitive to varying that assumption; as a result we have greater confidence in the study's conclusions.

Results That Are Insensitive to Assumptions

In a cost-effectiveness analysis of the use of cyclosporine in kidney transplantation, the following sensitivity analyses were reported:

"Increasing the annual cost of dialysis had little impact on the incremental cost-effectiveness ratios. If the annual cost of dialysis were actually $31,742, then using [cyclosporine] instead of [azathioprine] would cost $16,586 per additional life-year [as compared to $19,800] and $8,125 [as compared to $9,700] per additional graft-year. Varying the annual probability of retransplantation (5%–15%), the first-year graft survival of patients receiving retransplants, or avoiding discounting also had little effect on this cost-effectiveness ratio." (Simon 1986)

7.4 Conclusion

This chapter has examined two tools used to adjust the values obtained in a socioeconomic evaluation. Discounting is used to account for the positive value of time preference; that is, costs and consequences incurred in the present have greater value than those occurring in the future. Although there is general agreement among analysts that discounting should be employed, there is less agreement on the appropriate discount rate. Commonly, a rate of 3% to 5% is used. Sensitivity analysis is another technique that is well accepted among researchers. It is used in socioeconomic evaluations when there is uncertainty regarding the precise values of particular variables (including discount rates) and when the analyst wishes to test the sensitivity of the results to varying key assumptions in the analysis.

[2] An attack rate is a measure of the incidence of a disease in the population, but it does not specify a period during which the disease occurs.

8 Issues in Study Design

8.1 Introduction

The heart of every research study is its design. The study design is the structure within which research activity is carried out. It determines the type of data that are collected, the methods of data collection, how the data are analyzed, and the interpretation of the results.

In perusing socioeconomic evaluations, it is apparent that there is a wide variety of study design available. Some studies go to great lengths to document all costs and consequences carefully as they occur. Other studies use data that are available from existing records. Some studies observe groups of patients being treated in routine clinical settings while others are adjuncts to clinical studies involving extremely careful control of interventions and follow-up.

Why are there so many different study designs? We will see that the choice of a study design is determined by a number of factors. The most important factors are the objectives of the study (which may be determined by clients when a study is commissioned), the availability of data, the availability of resources (time, money, and personnel) to conduct the study, the availability of a study population, and the way in which the results will be used.

There are at least four major dimensions along which socioeconomic evaluations can be arrayed:

1. How consequences are measured
2. The temporal nature of the study, that is, whether data were collected prior to the study's beginning (retrospective) or during the study (prospective)
3. Whether the study employed an experimental, quasi-experimental, or an observational design, that is, whether the researcher introduced a treatment or simply observed what occurs in the clinical setting without intervening in the process
4. Whether subjects were randomized to treatment groups.

8.2 Measurement of Consequences

This first dimension has already been introduced. Chapter 3 began by stating that the ideal formulation of a socioeconomic evaluation would be to measure all costs and all benefits over all time across all alternatives. The realities of research, however, dictate that the scope of the problem be more narrowly defined so that only the major relevant costs and benefits are examined (as determined by the analyst in relation to the objective of the study) for a limited number of alternatives. The scope of the study is further constricted when we choose one of several study types.

As discussed earlier, there are four basic study types that take into account both costs and consequences: cost-minimization analysis, cost-benefit analysis, cost-effectiveness analysis, and cost-utility analysis. These study types are distinguished, in large part, by how consequences are measured and valued. Figure 8.1 illustrates these study types and describes the costs and consequences that are included in each. At the bottom of the figure are descriptions of specific study formulations.

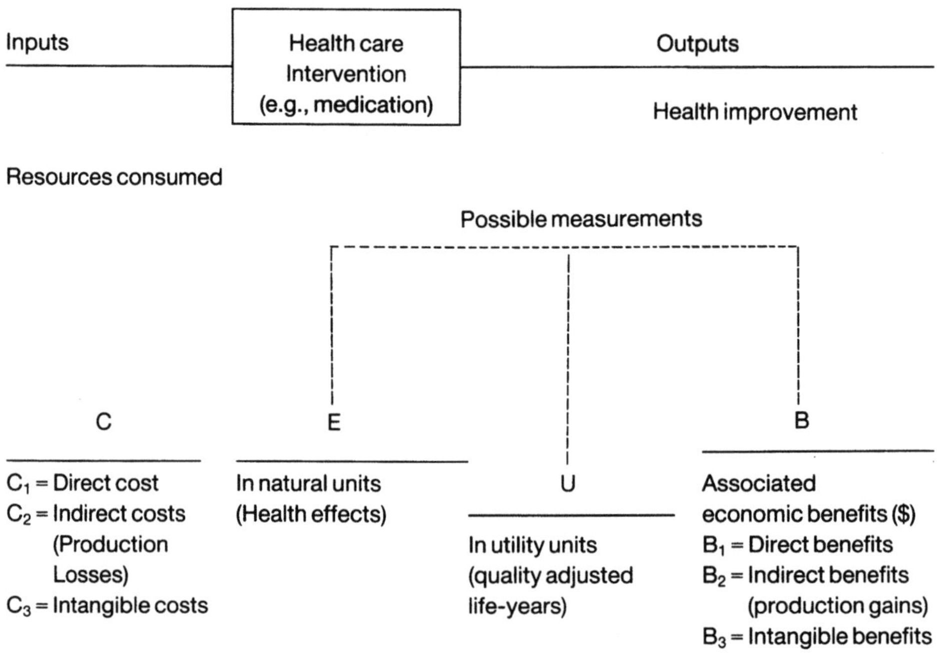

Common forms of analysis
1. Cost-minimization analysis (CMA): C_1; $C_1 + C_2$
2. Cost-benefit analysis (CBA): $B_1 + B_2 - C_1 - C_2$; $(B_1 + B_2)/C_1 + C_2)$
   Also sometimes includes consideration of C_3 and B_3.
3. Cost-effectiveness analysis (CEA): $(C_1 + C_2)/E$; $(C_1 - B_1)/E$; $(C_1 - B_1)/E + (C_2 - B_2)$
4. Cost-utility analysis (CUA): $(C_1 + C_2)/U$; $(C_1 - B_1)/U$; $(C_1 - B_1)/U + (C_2 - B_2)$

Fig. 8.1. Components of socioeconomic appraisal. (Adapted from Drummond et al. 1987)

8.3 Dimensions of Study Design

8.3.1 Prospective Studies

In a prospective study, interventions such as drugs are administered to patients (the *experimental group*) and the effects are recorded by study personnel. A comparison group that does not receive that particular intervention is called a *control group*. When patients are assigned randomly to the experimental and control groups, this is a *randomized controlled experimental design*. This type of design is most effective at controlling for potential biases that may enter into a study because of systematic differences between, for example, the severity of illness across the groups. If such *biases* were not controlled in some way, they would restrict our ability to say that the differences in observed effects between the two groups are actually caused by the intervention.[1]

Prospective Study:

A study in which data are collected during the study. One that follows a group of patients through time with perodic evaluations.

When applied to medications, this type of design is called a *randomized clinical trial (RCT)*. When neither the patient nor the health care provider know which group is receiving the intervention and which group is receiving an alternative therapy – typically a placebo or standard therapy – this is a randomized *double-blind* clinical trial. Double-blind RCTs are considered the best way to test the true effect of a drug and represent the ideal study design for the testing of medications. Randomization is a particularly important technique when researchers are uncertain about all the potential biases that may affect the outcome of a study. When researchers know that a particular variable, for example, the stage of cancer, will affect the outcome of testing a medication, then they will control for this variable explicitly, perhaps by entering patients with only one stage of cancer into the study or by examining the effects of the drug separately for patients with different stages of the disease.

Randomized Controlled Trial (RCT):

An experimental design in which subjects are randomized to one or more intervention groups and a control group.

By assigning patients randomly to separate groups, potential differences among patients are distributed to the two groups by chance. Some characteristics of patients are extremely important modifiers of the effect of medications. Depending on the issues examined, these may include the severity of the illness, patient age, gender, and the existence of complicating conditions (also called *co-*

[1] The most common biases which are controlled by the randomized experimental design are history, maturation, testing, statistical regression, selection, mortality, and instrumentation. These and other threats to the validity of a study are discussed at length in Campbell and Stanley (1963). Much of the following discussion is based on this text.

morbidities). These differences between patients are termed *confounders,* that is, they confound our ability to state unambiguously that A caused B. When patients are randomly assigned to treatment groups, these confounders are randomized as well, at least in theory. Under random assignment, chance will tend to distribute these important modifying characteristics equally to all groups. Of course, it is not possible to be certain that randomization was completely effective; therefore, results of studies should always be reported in terms of the *probability* that these results are true. (Chapter 13 discusses significance testing and probabilities.)

Socioeconomic Analysis in Conjunction with a Randomized Controlled Trial

A CBA was performed using data from a randomized controlled clinical trial of antibiotic prophylaxis for hysterectomy. In this study, 44 patients were randomly assigned to receive prophylaxis, while 42 patients were randomly assigned to a placebo group. The costs of caring for each of the two groups were compared and included the costs for the prophylactic antibiotic and the costs of treating infections that occurred in both groups. This study estimated that $492 was saved for each patient who received the prophylactic antibiotic for a vaginal hysterectomy, as compared with the alternative of no treatment. Because patients were randomly assigned to two groups, it was assumed that differences between the groups were attributable to the intervention, rather than to any uncontrolled biases. (Shapiro et al. 1983)

When random assignment is not used – for example, when the study drugs are administered to intact patient groups from separate hospitals – then it is likely that the groups will differ significantly along these characteristics. Patients from a teaching hospital may be more severely ill and they may have more coexisting illness than patients from a community hospital.

Although RCTs are normally required to test the effect of medications in order to obtain approval from regulatory agencies, they can also be the stage at which a socioeconomic evaluation is best performed. As the clinical trial is being conducted, researchers can simultaneously collect data on socioeconomic variables such as the utilization of medical resources, patients' quality of life, the utility of health states, and indirect costs.

Because RCTs control for biases and confounders, they have very high *internal validity*. Internal validity is the degree to which the results of a study are true for the group of subjects who participated in the study. When a study has high internal validity, we can say with a certain level of confidence that the effect seen in the intervention group is a result of the intervention and is not attributable to some other cause. In essence, internal validity deals with the causal relationship between the intervention and the observed effect.

External validity, however, is another matter. External validity is the extent to which the results of the study are generalizable to individuals outside the study. For decision-makers using the results of a socioeconomic evaluation, external validity is extremely important. The decision-maker is interested in how applicable these results are to other patients in other hospitals in other parts of the country. Without internal validity, the results of the study cannot be believed, but without external validity the results cannot be generalized beyond the setting of that particular study. It is in this respect that many RCTs suffer from a serious flaw that can make them a far less than ideal design for socioeconomic evaluations.

Several factors compromise the external validity of RCTs. First, the exclusion criteria for patients means that RCTs are usually conducted on highly selected patient groups. For example, young women of child-bearing age are generally excluded from RCTs of medications. Second, many RCTs are conducted in university medical centers which are not representative of the majority of clinical settings in which the drug will eventually be used. Third, the research protocol for an RCT often stipulates that additional testing be conducted on patients, or that the length of hospitalization be longer than routine for the condition of interest. These factors will distort the measures of resource utilization so that the costs of treatment and the sequelae of treatment may not be comparable in non-RCT settings. Because of these features of RCTs, decision-makers find it difficult to judge whether the results of a particular socioeconomic evaluation are applicable to the patient groups and settings in which they are interested.

The RCT is used by government regulatory agencies for assessing the *efficacy* of a medication, that is, the effects of the drug under ideal conditions. This does not necessarily reflect the use of the drug in normal clinical settings *(effectiveness)*. As a result, the clinical RCT is not always the ideal context for a socioeconomic evaluation and the randomized controlled trial is not always the ideal study design. Although the collection of economic data during RCTs is extremely useful and should be encouraged, it must be recognized that other study designs are acceptable as well and in some cases even preferable.

Not all prospective studies are RCTs. Indeed, RCTs are seldom used strictly for socioeconomic evaluations. A full discussion of prospective study designs is beyond the scope of this text; however, several of the more common designs will be briefly described. For the best contrast with the randomized experimental design, a pre-experimental design will be described first. This design is the weakest in terms of being able to attribute the effects of a study to the intervention, that is, it suffers from the most threats to internal validity.

8.3.2 Pre-test Post-test Design

A treatment may be tested by observing a single group of patients for some period of time under conditions of normal clinical practice and then administering the treatment to these same patients and observing any changes that occur. When there is only one group that is observed before and after treatment, this is a *pre-test post-test* design, also called a *one-group comparison* or a *within-patient* design. In effect, the patient population receiving the drug is acting as its own control.

Since this design does not entail randomization, it does not control for certain biases which, in turn, may limit our ability to say that observed changes are actually due to the intervention. For example, patients may take other treatments or the disease may follow some natural course of progression, either improvement or worsening. If this effect is not controlled, a treatment that actually slowed the worsening of a progressively debilitating disease may be judged ineffective when patients' health status appears to have declined between the before and after measurements.

Another explanation for changes in health status across two measurements on the same group is the effect of testing. The testing effect should be a particular concern when assessing health status or quality of life using questionnaires administered several times during the course of a study. The questions may themselves serve as a stimulus especially when the interval between testing is short. For example, consider a study that measures changes in quality of life before and after the administration of a medication. Patients are asked the same series of questions on two occasions regarding their social, physical, and emotional functioning. The initial administration of the questionnaire may sensitize patients to be more attentive to these aspects of their well-being. If there are no control group patients against whom to compare the study group responses, it is not possible unambiguously to ascribe differences between the pre-test and post-test scores to the medication. Another very common testing effect is the placebo response, the reaction to a compound or intervention that has no direct physiological action.

It is important for a reader to be aware of these potential pitfalls of the pre-test-post-test study design. A minimum standard for the author is to address these concerns to assure the reader that these potential threats to validity are minimized.

8.3.3 Quasi-experimental Designs

There are a number of study designs that do not meet the criteria of an experiment, but, if conducted well, can provide many of the benefits. Indeed, many quasi-experimental designs control for threats to external validity that remain dangers to the randomized experimental design. One commonly used type of quasi-experimental design is the *nonrandomized comparison group design.* Sometimes a study will employ two or more groups but patients are not randomly assigned to the groups. This happens, for example, when groups of patients at different hospitals participate in a study and each group receives a different treatment. The biggest danger in such a design is that the groups are not equivalent. Thus, this design has a control group, but it does not have randomization.

Quasi-experimental Design:

A study in which an intervention is introduced and its effect measured; however, there is no random assignment of subjects.

A bias that may be introduced in a quasi-experimental design is that differences between the two groups after treatment may have occurred as a result of different rates of dropout from the groups. For example, patients at one hospital may be less able to continue participating in a study for reasons not related to medical treatment. Although dropout rates may differ between the groups in an RCT, randomization tends to assure us that predisposing characteristics were not the cause of the differential dropout rates because these characteristics should have been distributed equally between the two groups.

One common way to minimize the problem caused by lack of random assignment is to use *statistical control.* It is possible to measure certain key characteristics of the people in the study groups. These characteristics would include factors that can potentially affect the outcome of interest, for example, age, gender, income, other illnesses, and medical or surgical complications. These factors are then included in multivariate statistical analyses (such as multiple regression) that control for the differences between groups. Basically, the groups are "equalized" according to these factors. The major limitation in such analyses is that some important characteristics may be omitted. Unmeasured differences between the groups may be the real causes of the outcomes. Statistical control is described in more detail later in this chapter under "Modeling" and in Chapter 14.

8.3.4 Variations on Prospective Studies

Regardless of whether a study is experimental or quasi-experimental, there are several common variations of prospective designs.[2] In a *parallel* design, two groups are each given a different treatment which they continue throughout the course of the study. This includes both randomized experimental designs or a non-randomized comparison group design.

```
         group A ---------
Parallel
         group B ---------
```

In a *crossover* design, each group is given a treatment (or one group is designated a control group), and at a later point in the study the groups switch treatments.

```
           group A ----\  /----
Crossover               \/
                        /\
           group B ----/  \----
```

The *time series* or *panel* design involves multiple observations of a single group over an extended period. An intervention is introduced at some point during the observation period so that there are multiple observations prior to the intervention and multiple observations after the intervention. There may be one or more interventions. Time series designs might be used to observe the effects of a contraceptive program in a population. Subjects not randomized; rather yearly birth rates are observed in a community for a period of time. The program is introduced into the community, and yearly birth rates are measured after the programm. Although this appears to be similar to the pre-test post-test design, the multiple observations before and after the intervention control for a number of important biases. Time series designs are often performed retrospectively, that is, using data already collected.

---

[2] For a more detailed description of these and other design refer again to the volume by Campbell and Stanley (1963).

The *separate sample pre-test-post-test* design is feasible to use when examining intact groups of subjects. In this design, subjects in one group are observed prior to an intervention, and subjects in another group are observed after an intervention.

Separate sample pre-test post-test	group A	---------	
	group B		---------

Another variant is the combined retrospective-prospective design. In this design, a treatment is administered to a group of subjects, the observations of the effect of the intervention are obtained prospectively, and these observations are compared with retrospective data.

8.3.5 Retrospective Studies

A retrospective study uses data that have been collected prior to the beginning of the current study. These data may be in the form of information collected during a previous study or the information may have been gathered simply for record-keeping purposes, such as medical records or insurance claims data. Retrospective studies are by definition all *observational studies,* that is, researchers observe what happens but they do not intervene or introduce a study factor or treatment.

Retrospective Study:

A study characterized by using data that have been collected prior to its beginning.

When a study uses *primary retrospective data,* the data have been collected by others prior to the beginning of this study; however, the data are not preselected or analyzed. Examples of this include the use of insurance claims files, hospital records, and work records.

Studies that use *secondary retrospective data* use information that has already been presented by other authors. For example, a study may use data for the rates of certain diseases or complications that are reported in previous studies.

A Study Using Secondary Data

This study examined the cost-effectiveness of preventing acute rheumatic fever by prophylactically using penicillin. Data for the analysis were obtained from published studies.

First, the alternative treatments and range of outcomes were described. Then the probabilities associated with each possible medical outcome were estimated using reports of other medical research studies. Finally, monetary costs were assigned using data from reports on the costs of medical services. (Tompkins et al. 1977)

Retrospective studies have several limitations. First, they are limited by the availability of data. Researchers using data from another study or from medical records have restricted information available to them. Previous studies may have ignored data on important confounding variables because the association was simply not known at that time. When data are used from natural sources such as hospital records, the researcher must be aware that the data may not be collected or recorded with the same rigor that applies to research studies; thus the reliability of the data may be suspect.

Second, retrospective studies are limited in the extent to which statements of causality can be made. In a retrospective study, researchers cannot be certain that the alleged cause preceded the alleged effect; thus, it is not possible to state that A *caused* B. A third limitation is the lack of randomization to an intervention and a control group. Any observed effects may be attributable to factors other than those studied.

Retrospective studies do have a number of advantages over prospective studies. First, when the condition is rare, it is possible to study fewer individuals than in a prospective study. By examining only those cases that have developed the disease, researchers are able to include fewer subjects. By matching cases with noncases (that is, patients with disease to those without disease), the researcher can study those factors that are present in the cases and absent in the noncases. An alternative retrospective design might use massive data sets such as insurance claims data bases to obtain information on rather rare conditions.

A second advantage of retrospective studies is that they are conducted in natural settings, that is, they are not subject to the biases that might be introduced when experiments are conducted. For example, when subjects know that they are being observed, their behavior may change. This is termed the "Hawthorne effect." Furthermore, because subjects are observed in natural settings, they may be more representative of the population, thus decreasing the likelihood of selection bias. Natural settings tend to maximize external validity, or the generalizability of study findings. A third advantage of retrospective studies is that they may be less expensive and less time-consuming than prospective studies. Thus, information may be available more quickly and with a smaller investment of resources.

8.4 Modeling

Modeling studies seek to simulate processes that occur through time. They are useful ways of attempting to describe those factors which are important determinants of a certain phenomenon. Modeling often uses retrospective data and fairly sophisticated computer programs that operate on multiple variables simultaneously. (Decision analysis is a type of modeling study and is the topic of Chapter 11.)

Modeling:

An analytical technique used to simulate processes that occur through time; often used to explain the impact of numerous independent variables on one or more dependent variables.

Because it is not possible to manipulate an intervention or to employ randomization in retrospective studies, it is necessary to control for other possible factors that could have caused the effects that we observe. In the absence of a control group and randomization that would allow us to state with a reasonable degree of certainty that A caused B, researchers employ *statistical control.* The most common statistical control method is regression analysis. In this method, multiple relevant factors thought to have an impact on the *dependent variable* of interest are examined in unison. The example shown below applies multiple regression analysis to control for confounders. This analytical process is discussed at length in Chapter 13.

A Retrospective Study Using Primary Data and Statistical Control

The cost-effectiveness of transdermal nitroglycerin (TDN) was compared with long-acting oral nitrates using Medicaid claims data. This involved a comparison of the use of medical resources by patients who were started on each of the drugs. There were significant differences between the groups in their severity of illness as measured by previous myocardial infarctions and use of other medications. In order to control for these confounders, the authors used multiple regression, incorporating pretreatment levels of resource use, patient demographic characteristics, and diagnosis of hypertension or heart failure as predictors of resource use after treatment. (Huse et al. 1988)

In essence, this study attempts to mimic a randomized controlled trial by equalizing the comparison groups in terms of the important modifiers and then observing the effects of the intervention. Where the RCT uses randomization to equalize the study groups, this study utilized statistical control to achieve the same effect. The extent to which this is successful depends on two factors. First, the researchers must have identified the correct confounders in order to truly equalize the groups. Any important modifiers that remain unidentified are not measured and, hence, are not statistically controlled.

Second, the confounders must have been operationalized correctly. *Operationalization* is the process whereby variables are defined in a way that can be measured. The variable must be defined appropriately, that is, the variable must be measuring what it purports to measure. For example, researchers might hypothesize that a new medication would result in so much improvement in patients' health that they were more likely to be discharged to their own homes rather than to an extended care facility. But the researchers knew that an important confounding variable, such as the patient's level of social support, may be an even stronger determinant of the discharge location of the patient. Thus, they decided to measure social support and they operationalized social support as marital status. Patients who were married were considered to have a high level of social support whereas patients who were single, widowed, or divorced had a low level of social support. It is very likely, however, that this operationalization of an important variable is not an accurate indicator of social support. For example, widowed patients living in the home of a child may have high levels of social support in reality, but appear to have low levels by this measure.

8.5 Conclusion

The randomized controlled trial (RCT) is the standard for evaluating the efficacy of medications, but there are several limitations to this study design that limit its applicability to socioeconomic evaluations. Most importantly, RCTs may suffer from problems of external validity, that is, they may not be generalizable. Nonetheless, the collection of socioeconomic data during RCTs can be extremely helpful in clarifying the quality of life and economic impact of a medication. A number of other prospective study designs are acceptable forms of socioeconomic analysis.

Retrospective studies (which utilize data collected prior to the beginning of the study) may utilize primary or secondary data. Modeling studies employ statistical control in order to assess the impact of a medication minus the effect of important confounders.

9 How to Assess a Socioeconomic Evaluation

9.1 Introduction

This chapter summarizes the information that has been presented in the previous chapters and outlines a process for evaluating reports of socioeconomic evaluations. Table 9.1 summarizes the major study types which have been discussed and differentiates them according to key parameters. This table provides a rudimentary guide to deciding which form of analysis is most appropriate for a given research problem.

The following outline should enable readers to assess a research report systematically. The answers to these questions will reveal the extent to which a study adheres to the most fundamental guidelines for socioeconomic evaluations. At the end of this chapter, several studies are analyzed using this outline.

9.2 Guide for Evaluating Socioeconomic Evaluations

Objective of the Study

What is the main research question?
Is more than one research question being considered?

Type of Study

What type of study is being performed?
- Cost-benefit analysis
- Cost-utility analysis
- Cost-effectiveness analysis
- Cost-minimization analysis
- Cost of illness study
- Quality of life study

Was this the most appropriate study type to use?
Is the study described actually what the authors purport it to be?

Table 9.1. Types of socioeconomic evaluation

Type of study	Intervention costs	Consequences	Measurement of consequences	Compares alternatives	Assumes equivalent effectiveness
Cost-benefit analysis	Monetary value of resources consumed	Monetary value of outcomes	Economic	Not necessarily although comp-risons are implicit	No
Cost-utility analysis	Monetary value of resources consumed	Utility of health effects	Quality adjusted life years (QALYs)	Yes	No
		Indirect costs	Economic		
		Subsequent use of resources	Economic		
Cost-effectiveness analysis	Monetary value of resources consumed	Effects on health	Lives saved	Yes	No
			Years of life saved		
		Indirect costs	Cases treated		
		Subsequent use of resources	Economic		
Cost-minimization analysis	Monetary value of resources consumed	Direct medical costs	Economic	Yes	Yes
Cost of illness study	Not applicable	Monetary value of resources consumed in treating illness	Economic	Not necessary	No
		Indirect costs	Economic		
Quality of life study	Disregarded	Impact on social, intellectual, psychological, physical and general well-being	Detailed questionnaires specific to the conditions being studied	Not necessary	No

Perspective

What is the perspective of the analysis?

- Society
- Third party payers
- Health care provider
- Patient

Is this the most appropriate perspective?
Does the perspective chosen ignore important costs or consequences?

Alternatives

The alternatives under consideration should be described in the study.
The following categories are helpful in understanding the alternatives being compared:
- Are the alternatives preventive, diagnostic, therapeutic, or research?
- Are they drugs, devices, surgical techniques, behavior change strategies (eg. education), or social welfare interventions?

Were any obvious interventions missed?
Was a "no treatment" alternative included, if appropriate?

Pathways of Clinical Management

Are the intervention inputs and outcomes fully described?

Costs

Which categories of cost were included?
- Direct medical (costs of supplying the medical services)
- Direct nonmedical (transportation, housekeeping, babysitting)
- Indirect (loss of productivity)

Valuation of costs:
- Were costs valued as market price (charges) or accounting costs?
- How were human costs valued? Willingness to pay? Human capital?

Do the costs reflect opportunity costs?
Are marginal costs or average costs addressed?
Are any obvious costs omitted?
Are hard-to-measure costs omitted?

Consequences

What types of consequences are described?
- Clinical outcomes, cases found, correct diagnoses, monetary?

How are consequences measured?
- Clinical consequences
  - Morbidity
  - Mortality
  - Use of health care resources
- Psychosocial consequences
  - "Intangibles": pain, suffering, anxiety
  - Quality of life:
    - What scales are used?

- Utility
    - How are utility values obtained?
    - Who are the respondents?
- Quality-adjusted life years

Economic consequences

- Use of health resources valued in economic terms (e.g., expenditures for medical services)
- Productivity (wages)
- Effects on other segments of the economy

What are the data sources?

- Primary or secondary

What is the evidence for effectiveness of the intervention?

Discounting

Was it performed?
What was discounted?
What rate(s) was (were) used?
What effect did discounting have on the results?

Sensitivity Analysis

Was it performed?
On what variables? That is, what assumptions were being tested?
What ranges were used?
What justification was given for these ranges?
Were findings sensitive to changes in values?

Research Design

Were primary or secondary data used?
Was it a prospective or a retrospective study?

- RCT, quasi-experiment, observational, modeling

Were the groups comparable?

- If not, was potential bias controlled for?

Results

Are these conclusions justifiable?
Are the results comparable to other studies?
How generalizable are the results?
Are noneconomic (e.g., ethical or distributional) issues addressed?
Was on overall measure of net benefit presented?

This guide may be used to assess any socioeconomic evaluation; however, not all questions can be answered for each study. For example, a cost-of-illness study will have no information on the consequences of an intervention and a quality of life study will not examine costs. This guide provides an outline of the most important issues to consider. The following case studies illustrate the use of the guide.

9.3 Case Study 1

An Economic Analysis of Parenteral Cephalosporins (Eisenberg et al. 1984)

Objective of the Study

What is the main research question?
  What savings can be expected in the hospital operating costs associated with once-daily antibiotics compared with those administered three to four times per day?
Is more than one research question being considered?
  This study also examined the cost impact of different types of treatment personnel and different technologies.

Type of Study

What type of study is being performed?
  Cost-minimization analysis.
Was this the most appropriate study type to use?
  This study type was appropriate because all clinical evidence available indicated that the efficacy of the once-daily and three or four times daily cephalosporins was equivalent for a wide variety of clinical conditions. Thus there was no need to examine the clinical effects.
Is the study described actually what the authors purport it to be?
  This study was described as possibly being a cost-effectiveness analysis but no effectiveness data were examined. It was also suggested that it might be a cost-benefit analysis. However, because only input costs were examined and no benefits were counted, it is more appropriately termed a cost-minimization study.

Perspective

What is the perspective of the analysis?
  That of the health care provider, specifically the hospital.
Is this the most appropriate perspective? Does the perspective chosen ignore important costs or consequences?

Given the research question posed, this is the most appropriate perspective. However, this narrow perspective ignores a wide range of costs and consequences. Nonetheless, it is likely that incorporating these costs would only reinforce the conclusions drawn from this study, that is, that additional cost savings would be demonstrated.

The authors identify several other perspectives that could be taken if other research questions were addressed. A study which examined the potential savings that might occur through early discharge from the hospital and use of this drug on an outpatient rather than inpatient basis would take the perspective of the third party payer. The perspective of society would entail examining the indirect costs associated with patients being able to return to work earlier.

Alternatives

The alternatives under consideration should be described in the study.

The alternatives examined were two frequently employed cephalosporins which were administered three to four times daily compared with a new drug that required only once daily administration.

Were any obvious interventions missed?

Because this study had a narrowly defined research question which dealt solely with the operating costs associated with different frequencies of antibiotic administration, other interventions were irrelevant.

Was a "no treatment" alternative included, if appropriate?

It was not appropriate because this drug was used only for patients who had severe infections.

Pathways of Clinical Management

The intervention inputs and outcomes should be fully described.

The study report went into considerable detail outlining the pathway of clinical management relevant to the cost accounting procedure. In addition, because this was a prospective study, actual work steps could be observed. This process first entailed defining a detailed flowchart which diagramed the processes required to administer the antibiotics. Then time-and-motion methods were used to observe hospital staff activities involved in preparing, dispensing, and administering the drug and attending the lines. Study team members recorded the amount of time spent in each activity, the level of personnel involved, and the supplies utilized at each stage.

Costs

Which categories of costs were included?

Direct medical (costs of supplying the medical services)

The authors computed average variable administration costs per dose (including personnel and materials costs) and did not include the costs of the drug itself. Considerable effort was expended in distinguishing fixed from variable costs when describing the pathways of clinical management because only variable costs would change with different dosing frequencies. Fixed costs, including overheads, could be ignored because these costs are invariate with respect to dosing frequency.

Direct nonmedical (transportation, housekeeping, babysitting)

Not included.

Indirect (loss of productivity)

Not included.

Valuation of costs: Were costs valued as market price (charges) or accounting costs?

Personnel costs were estimated using hourly wage rates which were averaged and weighted by the actual personnel hours involved in performing the activity. Material costs were estimated by using purchasing information.

How were human costs valued? Willingness to pay? Human capital?

Indirect costs were not included.

Do the costs reflect their opportunity costs?

Yes. The detailed cost-accounting procedure identified the opportunity costs of the services from the perspective of the hospital.

Are marginal costs or average costs addressed?

Because this study focused on the difference in costs between antibiotics administered once versus three to four times daily, marginal costs were addressed.

Are any obvious costs omitted? Are hard to measure costs omitted?

The cost accounting procedure was very thorough.

Consequences

No consequences were examined; it was assumed that the alternative regimens had equivalent efficiency.

Discounting

Discounting was not necessary because the scope of the study covered a very short period and no costs were deferred.

Sensitivity Analysis

Was it performed?

Resource use was measured directly through observation at four hospitals during a 2-week period across all three work shifts and averaged across the observations. Results were reported separately across institutions. As a result, there was less uncertainty about these values than if fewer data points had been obtained or if secondary data were used. Thus, sensitivity analysis was not imperative.

Research Design

Were primary or secondary data used?

This study entailed the collection of primary data.

Was it a prospective or a retrospective study?

Data were collected in a prospective fashion.

RCT, quasi-experiment, observational, modeling?

It was an observational study.

Were the groups comparable? If not, was potential bias controlled?

There was an implicit assumption that patients receiving the once daily antibiotic would not differ from those receiving the three or four times daily antibiotic in any way that would change the variable costs associated with the administration of the drugs. This assumption is justified if the drugs are truly comparable in clinical effectiveness and would be employed with the same type of patients.

Results

This study reported costs per dose for four different hospitals and for several methods of preparing and administering antibiotics. It was calculated that using the once daily antibiotic would result in $5.42 average savings per patient day. This amounted to an average savings of $155 per bed per year. More than half the savings resulted from lower material costs.

Are these conclusions justifiable?

The conclusions are consistent with the calculations presented. These figures do not include the costs of the antibiotic and are based on the assumption of equivalent efficacy of antibiotics regardless of dosing frequency. If these factors are not salient to the relative costs of the dosing regimens, then the conclusions about the cost savings associated with the once daily drug are warranted. The conclusions regarding the cost savings inherent in a once daily regimen are contingent on the assumption that the time "saved" will be, in turn, "spent" on other activities which are useful to the organization; however, a scenario can be imagined in which the "saved" time would be absorbed in taking more time for fewer tasks. The authors address this assumption by also examining nursing costs as a fixed cost and show that savings decrease by approximately 40%.

Are the results comparable to those of other studies?

The authors reported a similar study performed 5 years earlier which examined fixed and variable costs per drug dose. The results of this study were consistent with those of the earlier study.

How generalizable are the results?

This study paid particular attention to differences in drug therapy practices between hospitals, such as differences in personnel mix, supplies, and technology. Because detailed cost results were presented for multiple practice situations, the results should be generalizable to a wide spectrum of settings.

Are noneconomic (e.g., ethical or distributional) issues addressed?

Because of the perspective, this study was solely concerned with identifying methods to lower hospital costs of administering antibiotics.

Was an overall measure of net benefit presented?

Only input costs were measured.

9.4 Case Study 2

A Comparison of Treatment for Prostatic Cancer (Henriksson and Edhag 1987)

Objective of the Study

What is the main research question?

What are the costs and medical consequences associated with estrogen therapy versus orchidectomy for prostatic cancer patients?

Is more than one research question being considered?

No.

Type of Study

What type of study is being performed?

This is a cost-effectiveness analysis comparing the costs per case treated, and presenting results for orchidectomy-treated cases, all estrogen-treated cases, estrogen-treated cases without complications, and estrogen-treated cases with complications.

Was this the most appropriate study type to use?

A CUA may have shed light on the psychosocial impact of the two treatments by taking into account patients' valuations of orchidectomy as well as the complications of estrogen therapy. For example, patients may have considered orchidectomy so disagreeable that estrogen therapy, even with its higher risk of complications, may have been preferable from the patient's point of view.

Is the study described actually what the authors purport it to be?

Yes. Although the authors do not explicitly present their results as costs per case treated, this is a cost-effectiveness analysis.

Perspective

What is the perspective of the analysis?

The perspective appears to be that of a third party payer because all medical costs which would be relevant to an insurance company or a national sickness fund were included. Because indirect costs and psychosocial consequences were not included, the societal perspective was not taken.

Is this the most appropriate perspective? Does the perspective chosen ignore important costs or consequences?

This study did not take the perspective of the patient, which would have required assessing each therapy's impact on quality of life. Such information may have been a potent determinant of the acceptability of each therapy.

Alternatives

The alternatives under consideration should be described in the study.

Estrogen therapy is described in some detail, including dosage of both the oral and intramuscular preparations. Both alternatives are palliative modalities in the treatment of cancer; one is a medication and the other is surgery.

Were any obvious interventions missed?

Two commonly used forms of treatment are radical retropubic prostatectomy (for localized tumors) and irradiation (for more widespread cancers). The impact on the analysis of ignoring these forms of therapy is unclear.

Was a "no treatment" alternative included, if appropriate?

A no treatment alternative was not appropriate for these cancer patients.

Pathways of Clinical Management

The intervention inputs and outcomes should be fully described.

The medical resources required to provide cancer therapy, follow-up, and treatment of complications seem to be fully described. In addition, the medical complications resulting from the treatments are portrayed. No mention was made of any surgical complications in the orchidectomy group.

Costs

Which categories of cost were included?

Only the direct medical costs associated with inpatient, outpatient, and drug therapy were included. This included costs of surgery, costs of drugs, one radiation treatment of the breasts for estrogen patients, emergency room visits, office visits, subsequent hospitalizations, and treatment of complications from surgery and from estrogen.

Direct nonmedical (transportation, housekeeping, babysitting)

Not included.

Indirect (loss of productivity)

Not included.

Valuation of costs:

Were costs valued as market price (charges) or through actual accounting (i.e., an attempt to measure true economic cost)?

No information was provided regarding how resource costs were valued.

How were human costs valued? Willingness to pay? Human capital?

No indirect costs were examined.

Is the concept of opportunity cost addressed?
No.
Are marginal costs or average costs addressed?
This study examines average costs.
Are any obvious costs omitted? Are hard to measure costs omitted?
If nonmedical costs (such as transportation costs and patient time) had been incorporated into the analysis, the disparity between the two treatments would have been even wider because of the monthly visits required for estrogen injections. Because the sources for monetary values are not indicated, it is unclear whether all necessary costs are included.

Consequences

What types of consequences are described?
This study measured both clinical (side effects of the treatments) and cost (medical resource use) consequences associated with each therapy.
How are consequences measured?
Clinical consequences are measured as morbidity resulting from side effects from estrogen therapy (myocardial infarction, congestive heart failure, angina pectoris, cerebral infarction, intermittent claudication, and deep vein thrombosis), mortality resulting from estrogen therapy (myocardial infarction), and mortality resulting from prostatic cancer. No psychosocial consequences (quality of life, utility) are assessed. Use of health care resources is measured in monetary terms rather than in the number of resources used.
What are the data sources?
Data were collected during a clinical trial.
What is the evidence for effectiveness of the intervention?
This study was conducted as part of a clinical trial; thus, medical effectiveness data were obtained concurrently with resource use.

Discounting

Discounting was not necessary because all events occurred within a one-year period.

Sensitivity Analysis

No sensitivity analyses were performed; nonetheless, there are a number of uncertainties which are not addressed in this study. First, the authors state that a one-year follow-up to examine the relative efficacy of the two antitumor therapies is probably not long enough to state with assurance that their efficacy is similar. A difference in efficacy between the therapies could change the results of the analysis. Second, no data are provided regarding the sources or generalizability of cost information. Third, it is assumed that the complication rate for estrogen therapy will continue at the same rate as witnessed during the first year. Sensitivity analysis could address the uncertainty inherent in these estimates.

Research Design

Were primary or secondary data used?
Primary data from a randomized trial were used.
Was it a prospective or a retrospective study? RCT, quasi-experiment, observational, modeling?
The study was a prospective randomized trial of two therapies.
Were the groups comparable? If not, was potential bias controlled?
Patient groups were comparable with respect to demographic characteristics and cardiovascular risk factors.

Results

The average cost per case treated with orchidectomy was 32 162 SEK (Swedish Crowns). Average cost per case treated with estrogen therapy was 28 228 SEK. The difference was 3 934 SEK. The cost of treating a patient who received estrogen therapy but who experienced complications was 54 303 SEK. Yearly costs of estrogen therapy were 2 500 SEK. This means that 2½ years of estrogen therapy are equivalent in cost to orchidectomy. The authors suggest that if the estrogen group continues to have a higher complication rate the differential in costs could become even smaller and could quickly favor orchidectomy.
Are these conclusions justifiable?
Because significant economic and psychosocial costs were not examined and because of uncertainty regarding some key variables (long-term efficacy and complication rates associated with the treatments and the method of valuing costs), the results are incomplete.
Are the results comparable to those of other studies?
The results of other studies are not discussed for comparison.
How generalizable are the results?
The generalizability of this study is limited given the relatively short follow-up time, the lack of information regarding the occurrence of future complications, the lack of data regarding how cost estimates were generated, and the failure to take into account indirect and psychosocial costs.
Are noneconomic (e.g., ethical or distributional) issues addressed?
No.
Was an overall measure of net benefit presented?
No.

Part II

Technical Aspects

10 Quality of Life Assessment in Socioeconomic Evaluations[1]

For most patients with chronic disease, it is often not possible to eliminate or cure their illness. The goal of treatment is improved functioning through a reduction in the symptoms or the severity of an illness, or the limitation of disease progression (Wenger et al. 1984). In this case, there may be a direct relationship between functional improvement due to the therapeutic intervention and changes in the quality of life. Despite the effectiveness of some therapies in eliminating symptoms of disease, some clinically effective therapies also create residual limitations in functional ability. The evaluation of new therapies requires a more complete understanding of the impact of the treatment on the patient's physical, social, and psychological status. This combination of social, functional, and behavioral outcomes, or total psychosocial and physical well-being, is called *quality of life.*

10.1 Definition of Quality of Life

Quality of life is a multidimensional concept that encompasses the physical, emotional, and social effects of an illness or treatment (see Table 10.1). There are five main dimensions of quality of life: physical functioning, psychological functioning, social functioning, cognitive functioning, and general well-being.

Table 10.1. Dimensions of quality of life

Dimension	Examples
Physical functioning	Mobility, self-care, ability to perform activities of daily living, pain, physical symptoms
Psychological functioning	Depression, anger, anxiety, helplessness, expectations about the future
Social functioning	Participation in social activities, sexual functioning, Family relationship, recreational activities
Cognitive functioning	Memory, alertness, judgement
General well-being	General health, perceptions, life satisfaction

[1] Contributed by Dennis A. Revicki, PhD, Senior Research Scientist, Battelle Medical Technology and Policy Research Center, Washington, DC.

Quality of life includes a broad range of functional limitations, capabilities, and perceptions that may influence an individual's performance, satisfaction with life, and well-being. In assessing quality of life is it important to consider not only the actual functional capability, but also the individual's perceptions of the impact of this ability or disability on his or her life. Subjective as well as objective indicators are required for a comprehensive evaluation of quality of life.

Changes in quality of life as a result of exposure to a new therapy may be positive or negative. In many cases, there may be no clear advantage for one therapy compared with another across all dimensions of quality of life. Rather, there is often a profile of effects on different dimensions. Positive effects may be due to a reduction in symptoms, increased functional ability, or improved perception of well-being. Conversely, negative effects on life quality may arise if the treatment causes additional symptoms, decreases functional capability, or reduces sense of well-being because of adverse effects of the therapy. Even though there may be considerable evidence for the clinical efficacy of a new therapy, it may not be prescribed by physicians or may not be well tolerated in patients unless it does not adversely affect quality of life or those dimensions of quality of life that are important to the patient.

The addition of quality of life measures to clinical trials for new drugs or medical devices assists in characterizing the advantages and disadvantages of alternative, competing therapies. Quality of life assessment is most useful in situations where:

1. There are slight differences in patient survival between the alternative therapies under comparison
2. There are a number of equally effective therapies for a specific chronic disease or condition
3. The therapy is effective in decreasing mortality but is fairly toxic, leading to additional morbidity
4. The therapy is lifelong, the disease complication rate is low, and patients are asymptomatic or only mildly symptomatic (Wenger et al. 1984)
5. Comparisons are being made across healthcare programs having differing implications for mortality and morbidity

Understanding the impact of a therapy on the patient's physical, psychological, and social functioning may help decision-makers, physicians, and their patients evaluate the benefits of various competing therapeutic regimens.

For asymptomatic conditions, a therapeutic intervention may be very effective, but concerns about quality of life may discourage its use. Although there may be physiological changes (for example, lowered blood pressure, decreased serum cholesterol) associated with a drug treatment, patients often do not perceive any concomitant change in their health or psychological well-being. Indeed, the drug's side effects may reduce a patient's well-being. There are practical and ethical reasons for examining quality of life in patients treated for asymptomatic conditions. A therapy must be demonstrated to have no impact or minimal impact on quality of life to insure that patients are not placed at additional risk over and above that expected from the condition itself.

For example, a new drug may be demonstrated to be effective and safe in reducing total serum cholesterol; however, it will not reduce the incidence of cardiovascular disease in patients with hypercholesterolemia unless it is prescribed by physicians and accepted by patients. This acceptance may, in part, be determined by the drug's effect on the patient's quality of life. For asymptomatic conditions, such as hypercholesterolemia and mild hypertension, physicians may be reluctant to increase doses even when the condition is not yet under control unless there is sufficient evidence on the effects of the therapy on quality of life. Physician behavior may be due to their genuine concern that higher doses may produce adverse effects that reduce the patient's overall physical or psychological well-being even if the drug is clinically effective.

Patients may also be overly cautious about treatment for an asymptomatic condition. Some hypertensive patients view the use of medication to be more troubling than their relatively symptomless disease, resulting in noncompliance and ineffective long-term treatment (Croog et al. 1986). Valid and reliable information on the effects of alternative therapies on quality of life may increase physician and patient confidence in a therapy and may increase patient compliance and the benefits of the treatment.

10.2 Importance of Quality of Life Assessment

Quality of life and functional health status are emerging as important measures for evaluating the outcome of health care interventions for chronic disease. Three conferences have recently been held on these topics to clarify conceptual issues and examine different methods for measuring quality of life (Katz 1987; Lohr and Ware 1987; Lohr 1989). The parmaceutical industry is currently supporting a number of studies designed to examine potential quality of life effects associated with alternative drug therapies for cancer, anemia, diabetes mellitus, hypertension, and arthritis (Luce et al. 1989). There is every indication that interest in incorporating quality of life assessments into clinical trials is increasing among members of the pharmaceutical industry (Luce et al. 1988).

Health administrators and medical care providers need to understand the effects of different therapies on quality of life in order to make decisions about alternative treatments for illness. Quality of life information is particularly important when a number of equally effective therapies are available for a specific disease. For example, although different antihypertensive drugs are effective in reducing blood pressure, there are significant differences in their effects on patient quality of life (Croog et al. 1986; Revicki and Underwood 1988). Selecting the best antihypertensive drug for a patient may involve decisions about potential effects on quality of life as well as the control of hypertension. A drug that is effective in reducing blood pressure but which creates difficulties for the patient in terms of sleep disturbances and decrease in general well-being may not be taken or may lead to patient dissatisfaction with the physician.

10.3 Measurement of Quality of Life

A number of different methods are available for measuring quality of life including both generic and disease-specific measures. Several recently published books provide excellent introductions to this area as well as summaries of the available measures (Walker and Rosser 1988; McDowell and Newell 1987). Among the most widely used general health status measures are the Sickness Impact Profile (Bergner et al. 1987), the Quality of Well-Being Scale (Bush 1984), the McMaster Health Index Questionnaire (Chambers 1988), and the General Health Rating Index (Brook et al. 1979). For example, the Sickness Impact Profile assesses illness-related dysfunction in physical function (that is, ambulation, mobility, body care, and movement), psychosocial function (that is, social interaction, alertness behavior, emotional behavior, communication), and independent categories of work, eating, sleep and rest, home management, and recreation and pastimes. Specific examples of questions from quality of life scales are included at the end of this chapter.

Most of the general measures assess several quality of life dimensions and are therefore quite lengthy. Short forms are available for the General Health Rating Index (Stewart et al. 1988) and the Sickness Impact Profile for patients with low back pain (Roland and Morris 1983). In addition, there are a number of short scales that are designed to measure only one or a limited number of quality of life dimensions, such as the Center for Epidemiologic Studies Depression scale (Radloff 1977) and the Activities of Daily Living Scale (Katz and Akpom 1976). The selection of the measures for a quality of life study depends upon the purpose of the investigation, the suspected quality of life effects of the treatment, attributes of the study population, the psychometric characteristics of the measures, and resource limitations.

Although not explicitly discussed in most quality of life studies, the identification of measures can be determined by developing a theoretical model, based on existing research evidence, concerning the probable relationship between the therapy of interest and patients's social, physical, and psychological functioning. This list of potential benefits and adverse effects can then be used to select the relevant dimensions of quality of life and the scales for measuring these dimensions. The specific scales are chosen based on the match between their content and the objective of the study, their psychometric characteristics (that is, reliability, validity, sensitivity to change), and aspects of their mode of administration (for example, respondent burden, clarity, self-report versus interview).

Example of a Quality of Life Study

This study examined the quality of life effects of three antihypertensive drugs (i.e., captopril, propranolol, methyldopa). A number of measures of different quality of life dimensions were selected that were throught to be affected by drug treatment for high blood pressure. These included measures of: a) general well-being, b) sleep dysfunction, c) sexual problems, d) work performance, e) social activity participation, f) physical distress, and g) cognitive function.

The measures of quality of life were administered three times over a 12-month period to hypertensive patients on the three treatment regimens. The investigators found that there were significant differences in various aspects of quality of life despite comparable efficacy of the drugs in decreasing blood pressure.
There were no differences between the treatment groups on measures of sleep dysfunction, social participation, and visual memory. The captopril group had higher scores on measures of general well-being and physical distress symptoms compared with the propranolol and methyldopa groups. The findings of this study demonstrate that different antihypertensive drugs have different effects on quality of life and that these effects can be measured with existing techniques (Croog et al. 1986).

10.4 Conclusion

The pharmaceutical industry is continuing to support the inclusion of quality of life measures into randomized clinical trials of recently developed drugs. The results of quality of life studies will be used to demonstrate the relative advantages and disadvantages of one treatment compared with another for the same indication. Additional information concerning the effects of different drugs on physical, psychological, and social functioning will be useful to physicians, health administrators, insurers, and other health care decision-makers. The judicious use of these studies may assist physicians in identifying the quality of life implications associated with the prescription of a particular therapy.

Health care professionals are increasingly convinced that one of the major objectives of medical care is the enhancement of quality of life rather than the cure of disease or prolonged survival. The development of numerous life-saving medical technologies and their adoption by the health care system requires the evaluation of whether these new technologies improve the quality of life of their recipients as well as increase their survival. The combination of biomedical and quality of life outcome measures in randomized clinical trials of new medical technologies will provide physicians and health care decision-makers with sufficent information to compare alternative therapies for specific medical conditions or illnesses. In this way, judgments regarding the use of alternative treatments can be made based on the clinical efficacy and impact of the therapy on the patient's physical, social, and psychological status. Information on quality of life will assist physicians and their patients and patient's families in selecting treatments that alleviate disease and improve, or maintain, functional capacity and well-being.

10.5 Examples of Quality of Life Scale Items

The following questions have been drawn from several commonly used scales which measure quality of life. The questions have been selected to represent the five main areas which comprise quality of life and are presented in the format used in the questionnaires.

10.5.1 Social Functioning

PLEASE RESPOND TO (CHECK) ONLY THOSE STATEMENTS THAT YOU ARE SURE DESCRIBE YOU TODAY AND ARE RELATED TO YOUR STATE OF HEALTH.

1. I am going out less to visit people. _____
8. I am avoiding social visits from others. _____
16. I isolate myself as much as I can from the rest of the family. _____
19. I am not doing the things I usually do to take care of my children or family. _____

(from the *Sickness Impact Profile*)

10.5.2 Physical Functioning

4. At present, are you physically able to walk out-of-doors by yourself when the weather is good?
   1 NO → b
   2 YES → a

a. What is the farthest you can walk by yourself?
   1. ONE MILE OR MORE
   2. LESS THAN 1 MILE BUT MORE THAN 30 FEET (ABOUT THE SIDE OF A HOUSE)
   3. LESS THAN 30 FEET

b. Are you able to walk by yourself?
   4. BETWEEN ROOMS
   5. ONLY WITHIN A ROOM
   6. CAN'T WALK AT ALL

(from the *McMaster Health Index Questionnaire*)

10.5.3 Emotional Functioning

This section of the examination contains questions about how you feel and how things have been going with you. For each question check the answer which best applies to you.

7. I felt downhearted and blue DURING THE PAST MONTH.
   [ ] None of the time
   [ ] A little of the time
   [ ] Some of the time
   [ ] A good bit of the time
   [ ] Most of the time
   [ ] All of the time

(from the *Psychological General Well-Being Schedule*)

10.5.4 Intellectual Functioning

Often people's health affects the way they feel about life. For the next questions, please circle the choice that is closest to the way you feel about each statement.

	Strongly agree				Strongly disagree
16. I am a quick thinker.	1	2	3	4	5
21. I would say I nearly always finish things once I start them.	1	2	3	4	5
26. I am usually alert.	1	2	3	4	5

(from the *McMaster Health Index Questionnaire*)

10.5.5. General Well-being

This section of the examination contains questions about how you feel and how things have been going with you. For each question check the answer which best applies to you.

9. How happy, satisfied, or pleased have you been with your personal life? (DURING THE PAST MONTH)
   [ ] Extremely happy – could not have been more satisfied or pleased
   [ ] Very happy most of the time
   [ ] Generally satisfied – pleased
   [ ] Sometimes fairly happy, sometimes fairly unhappy
   [ ] Generally dissatisfied, unhappy
   [ ] Very dissatisfied or unhappy most or all of the time

(from the *Psychological General Well-being Schedule*)

Further Reading

Bergner MB, Bobbitt RA, Carter WB, Gilson BS (1987) The sickness impact profile: development and final revision of a health status measure. Med Care 19:787–805

Bombadier C, Ware J, Russell I, et al. (1986) Auranofin therapy and quality of life in patients with rheumatoid arthritis: results of a multicenter trial. Am J Med 81:565–578

Brook RH, Ware JE, Davies-Avery A, et al. (1979) Overview of adult health status measures fielded in Rand's Health Insurance Study. Med Care [Suppl] 17:1–131

Bush JW (1984) General Health Policy Model/Quality of Well-Being (QWB) Scale. In: Wenger NK, Mattson ME, Furberg CD, Elinson J (eds) Assessment of quality of life in clinical trials of cardiovascular therapies. Le Jacq, New York

Chambers LW (1988) The McMaster Health Index Questionnaire: an update. In: Walker SR, Rosser RM (eds) Quality of life: assessment and application. MTP Press, Lancaster

Croog SH, Levine S, Testa MA, et al. (1986) The effects of antihypertensive therapy on the quality of life. N Engl J Med 314:1657–1664

Evans R, Manninen D, Garrison L, et al. (1985) The quality of life of patients with end-stage renal disease. N Engl J Med 312:553–540

Katz S (ed) (1987) The Portugal conference: measuring quality of life and functional status in clinical and epidemiological research. J Chronic Dis 40:459–650

Katz S, Akpom CA (1976) Index of ADL. Med Care 14:116–118

Lohr KN (ed) (1989) Advances in health status assessment: conference proceedings. Med Care [Suppl] 27:51–5294

Lohr KN, Ware JE (eds) (1987) Proceedings of the advances in health assessment conference. Palm Springs, California 19–21 February 1986. J Chronic Dis 40:1s–191s

Luce BR, Weschler JM, Underwood C (1989) The use of quality-of-life measures in the private sector. In: Mosteller F, Falotico-Taylor J (eds) Quality of life and technology assessment, National Academy Press, Washington, DC

McDowell I, Newell C (1987) Measuring health: a guide to rating scales and questionnaires. Oxford University Press, New York

Najman JM, Levine S (1981) Evaluating the impact of medical care and technologies on the quality of life: a review and critique. Soc Sci Med 15:107–155

Radloff LS (1977) The CES-D scale: a self-report depression scale for research in the general population. Appl Psychol Measurem 1:385–401

Revicki DA, Underwood C (1988) Quality of life and non-insulin dependent diabetes mellitus. Battelle Human Affairs Research Centers, Washington

Roland M, Morris R (1983) A study of the natural history of back pain: development of a reliable and sensitive measure of disability in low-back pain. Spine 8:141–144

Stewart AL, Hays RD, Ware JE (1988) The MOS Short-Form General Health Survey: reliability and validity in a patient population. Med Care 26 (7):724–735

Walker SR, Rosser RM (eds) (1988) Quality of life: assessment and application. MTP Press, Lancaster

Wenger NK, Mattson ME, Furberg CD, Elinson J (eds) (1984) Assessment of quality of life in clinical trials of cardiovascular therapies. Le Jacq, New York

11 Decision Analysis

11.1 Definition of Decision Analysis

When decisions must be made in the face of uncertainty, decision analysis may be helpful. It is a quantitative analytical technique which describes a problem in terms of (a) multiple possible courses of action, (b) the probabilities that certain events and outcomes will occur, and (c) the value of the expected outcomes resulting from different courses of action. The principal goal of decision analysis is to determine the most appropriate course of action given the data available. When there is a great deal of uncertainty, it will often not be possible to identify an optimal strategy. In this case, decision analysis helps to structure a problem explicitly and rationally using the information that is available. Decision analysis has been used in socioeconomic evaluations as a means of quantifying the outcomes associated with various medical diagnostic modalities and treatments.

11.2 Bayes' Theorem

Decision analysis is based on Bayes' theorem, which asserts that the probability of B depends on the prior probability of A. For example, the probability of antibiotic B working in a certain patient is contingent on the probability of microorganism A being the cause of the infection. Bayes' theorem is represented by this formula:

$$P(B|A) = \frac{P(BA)}{P(A)}$$

This is read as "the probability of event B occurring given the fact that event A has occurred equals the probability of event B and event A occurring jointly divided by the probability of event A." This formula describes a condition called *statistical dependence,* that is, the occurrence of event B is contingent on the occurrence of event A.

Decision analysis is based on three different types of probability. *Prior probability* is the probability of an event before we have any new information about that event. *Conditional probability* is the probability of an event given that another event has occurred. *Posterior probability* is the revised probability of an event after new information has been obtained. "Prior" and "posterior" are used in reference to the new information which helps us to revise our probabilities.

Prior, Posterior, and Conditional Probabilities

A 67-year-old man with peripheral vascular disease is being evaluated for coronary heart disease (CHD). In the process of the evaluation, he received a thallium scan which turns out to be negative. The physician wants to know the probability of this man having CHD given the negative results on the scan, so the following table was constructed. The physician obtained the probability values in columns B and C from a review of the clinical literature.

A Diagnosis	B Prior probability of disease	C Conditional probability of negative scan	D Product (B × C)	E Posterior probability (100 × *D*/ sum of *D*)
Critical CHD	10%	5%	0.005	1.6%
Noncritical CHD	70%	20%	0.14	43.6%
Negligible CHD	20%	88%	0.176	54.8%

Before the scan was performed, the patient had a 10% probability of having critical coronary heart disease. After the negative scan, his probability of having critical disease reduced to 1.6%. Despite the negative scan results, however, he still has a nearly 50% chance of having some degree of CHD. (Pauker and Kassirer 1987)

11.3 Decision Trees

The primary tool of decision analysis is the *decision tree.* This is a diagram which illustrates all alternative courses of action in response to a specific problem. Figure 11.1 is a decision tree depicting whether or not to perform a pulmonary arteriogram on a patient with suspected pulmonary embolism. It begins at the left with a square *decision node* which indicates that a decision must be made at this point. This decision node is the point at which the physician decides whether or not to conduct an arteriogram. If an arteriogram is conducted, we reach a circle. This is called a *chance node;* at this point a chance event takes place. In this example, the patient has a particular probability of surviving the arteriogram and a particular probability of dying as a result of complications from the arteriogram. These probability values are depicted underneath the line representing each event. Probabilities are usually obtained from either a review of the clinical literature or from consultation with clinical experts.

At the far right hand side of the diagram lie all the possible outcomes that might occur as a result of the decisions and the chance events listed. Each outcome has an associated number called a *utility* listed in the ovals. Utilities are numbers that the researcher assigns to each outcome to represent the relative value of that out-

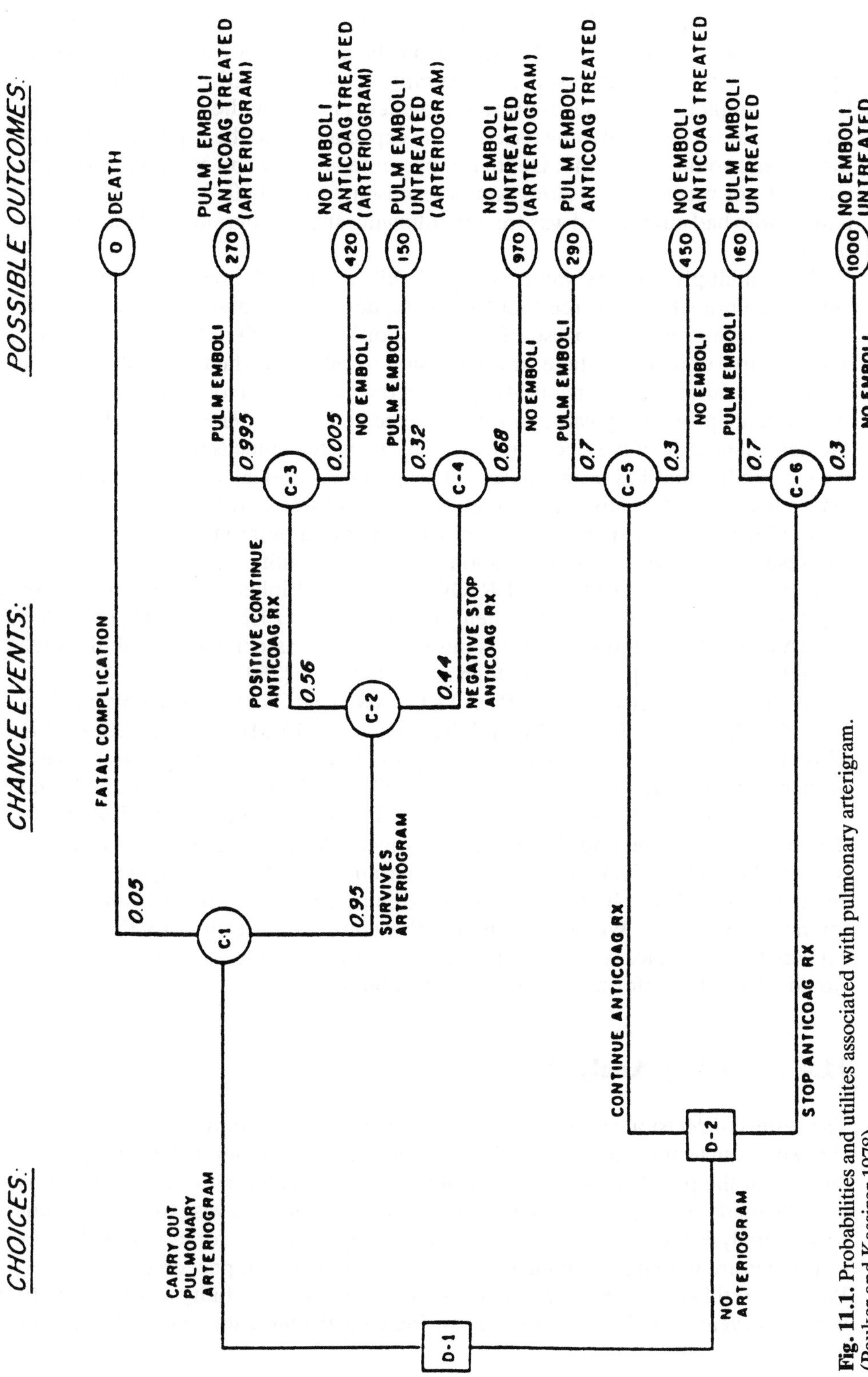

Fig. 11.1. Probabilities and utilites associated with pulmonary arterigram. (Pauker and Kassirer 1978)

come. For example, in a CEA there are two utility values: one monetary and one a measure of effectiveness. Utility values may be quality of life measures, morbidity events, or measures of resource consumption such as length of hospitalization. In this example, the utilities represent judgments made by the researchers of the relative value of each outcome based on life expectancy and the expected time that the patient would be healthy. Death is represented by zero; no emboli in a patient who did not receive an arteriogram is represented by 1000. The outcome of a patient who had emboli and was treated following an arteriogram received a utility of 270.

If we multiply a utility value by a probability value, the result is an *expected value*. The branch of the tree that has the highest expected value is the one that should be the preferred course of action. In order to reach a decision regarding which course of action to take, it is necessary to *fold back* the tree. Folding back is a process during which the utility associated with each outcome is multiplied by the proximal probability value to yield an expected value. (This process begins at the right-hand side of the decision tree.) This expected value is then multiplied by the probability that lies proximal to it. This process is repeated until we reach the choice between alternatives that lie at the left-hand side of the decision tree.

In Fig. 11.1, the expected utility of carrying out a pulmonary arteriogram ist the result of a series of computations. First, the utility of PULM EMBOLI ANTICOAG TREATED (ARTERIOGRAM) is multiplied by the probability of this event ($270 \times 0.995 = 269$). Then, the utility of NO EMBOLI ANTICOAG TREATED (ARTERIOGRAM) is multiplied by its associated probability ($420 \times 0.005 = 2$). These products are then added together ($269 + 2 = 271$). Next, the utility of PULM EMBOLI UNTREATED (ARTERIOGRAM) is multiplied by its probability ($150 \times 0.32 = 48$) and the utility of NO EMBOLI UNTREATED (ARTERIOGRAM) is multiplied by its probability ($970 \times 0.68 = 660$). These products are in turn added together ($48 + 660 = 708$). The new sums of 271 and 708 are the expected values for those nodes. This process continues until we reach the chance node depicting the chance outcomes after arteriogram. At this point, the expected value of carrying out an arteriogram is 440. Performing the same calculations on the lower half of the decision tree results in an expected value of 412 for no arteriogram. We would choose the course of action with the highest expected utility (since higher utilities signify more desirable outcomes); thus, we would choose to perform a pulmonary arteriogram.

11.4 Sensitivity Analysis

The results of decision analysis are only as valid as the probabilities and the utilities that we assign to specific choices, chance events, and outcomes. Often analysts are faced with the problem of having incomplete or uncertain data and assumptions must be made regarding certain values. In this situation, it is wise to perform sensitivity analysis (see Chap. 7). In sensitivity analysis, values for key probabilities or utilities are varied systematically in order to assess the impact on the outcome. Would we still choose the same course of action if the probability associated with a chance event were higher? Would varying a particular utility value change our decision? In essence, we are asking, "how robust are our results to changes in key variables?"

Researchers also use sensitivity analysis in order to define *threshold values.* These are values which represent cutoff or break-even points for our decisions. If values fall below this threshold value, we would choose not to follow a particular course of action. However, when values lie above the threshold, then we would choose that path.

A *one-way sensitivity analyisis* is performed when only one variable is changed. However, it is possible to vary multiple parameters at the same time. In a *Monte Carlo simulation,* all probabilities and utilities are allowed to vary simultaneously. This process requires a large number of calculations to identify the optimal decision. This is also called probabilistic sensitivity analysis.

11.5 Markov Processes

Decision trees are useful when examining clinical problems that occur over a relatively short period. However, conventional trees can become unwieldy when exploring options that occur within a long time frame, as is the case in most chronic diseases. In such situations, it is often useful to employ Markov models which describe cyclical changes in health states.

Markov models can replace decision trees or they may be grafted on to a decision tree at an appropriate point. A Markov model describes several discrete states of health in which a person may be at time 1. Then the model describes the possible states of health into which the person may move at time 2. Probabilities are associated with each change from one health state to another; these are termed *transitional probabilities.* This can continue ad infinitum until all people have moved through the model and have reached an end point such as death. Markov models are also called transition state models.

One major feature of Markov models is that the probabilities of moving from one state to another are independent of previous state changes. In other words, the model has no "memory" of previous states of health. This means that all subjects in the same health state have the same probability of moving to another state regardless of their prior transitions from one state to another. As in decision trees, probabilities are defined according to the clinical literature or based on expert opinion.

A Markov Model

In a study of the cost-effectiveness of cyclosporine in transplanting kidneys from cadavers, a Markov model was used. The following illustration depicts the model:

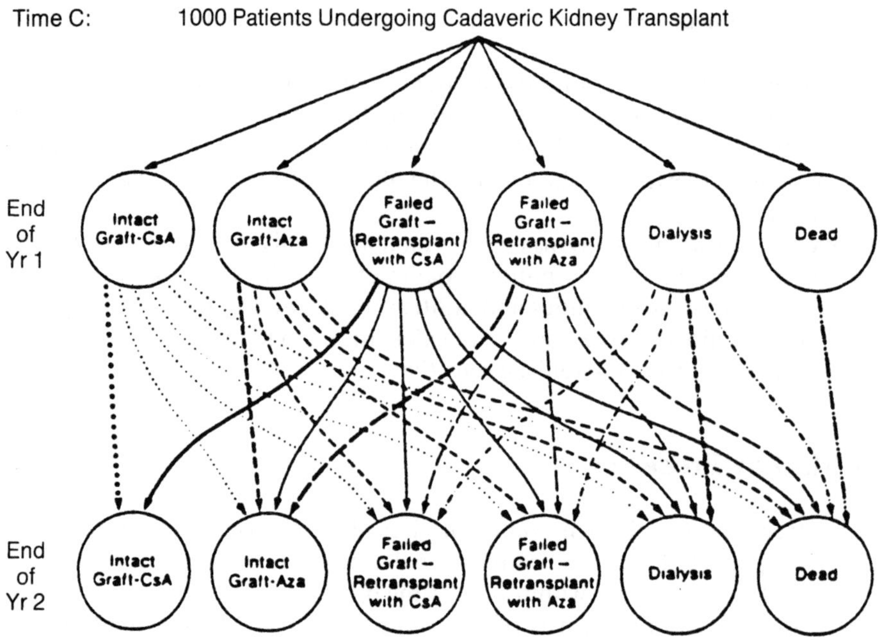

CsA refers to cyclosporine, Aza refers to azathioprine, both of which are immunosuppressive medications. Although no probability values are depicted in this model, each transition from one health state to another has an associated transitional probability.
Note that the first circle (Intact Graft-CsA) can result in six possible health state changes. These range from maintaining the same health state to death. The second circle (Intact Graft-Aza) can result in five different health states. The last circle (Dead) leads to only one health state (still Dead). All health states but Dead are termed "nonabsorbing" states; when no more transitions are possible, we have reached an "absorbing" state. (Simon 1986)

11.6 Conclusion

Decision analysis is a useful tool for socioeconomic evaluation. When data regarding the probability and utility values necessary for computation are available in the literature, decision analysis can be an efficient alternative to analysis and allows the researcher to explore the effects of changing key parameters and observing the effect of these changes on the choice of an optimal decision. However, the accuracy of the results obtained from decision analysis is contingent upon the accuracy of the data that are entered into the model. Often the probability values for particular chance events are unknown and utility values must be imputed on the basis of incomplete information.

Further Reading

Beck RJ, Pauker SG (1983) The Markov process in medical prognosis. Med Decis Making 3:419–458
Crane VS (1988) Economic aspects of clinical decision making: applications of clinical decision analysis. Am J Hosp Pharm 45:548–553
Doubilet P, Begg CB, Weinstein MC, Braun P, McNeil BJ (1985) Probabilistic sensitivity analysis using Monte Carlo simulation: a practical approach. Med Decis Making 5:157–177
Kassirer JP, Moskowitz AJ, Joseph L, Pauker SG (1987) Decision analysis: progress report. Ann Intern Med 106:275–291
McNeil BJ, Pauker SG (1984) Decision analysis for public health: principles and illustrations. Annu Rev Public Health 5:135–161
Pauker SG (1976) Coronary artery surgery: the use of decision analysis. Ann Intern Med 85:8–18
Pauker SG, Kassirer JP (1978) Clinical application of decision analysis: a detailed illustration. Semin Nucl Med 8:324–335
Pauker SG, Kassirer JP (1980) The threshold approach to clinical decision making. N Engl J Med 302:1109–1117
Pauker SG, Kassirer JP (1987) Decision analysis. N Engl J Med 316:250–258
Simon DG (1986) A cost-effectiveness analysis of cyclosporine in cadaveric kidney transplantation. Med Decis Making 6:199–205
Sox HC, Blatt MA, Higgens MC, Marton KI (1988) Medical decision making. Boston, Butterworth
Weiss JC, Melman ST (1988) Cost-effectiveness in the choice of antibiotics for the initial treatment of otitis media in children; a decision analysis approach. Pediatr Infect Dis J 7:23–26

12 Utility Analysis in Socioeconomic Evaluation

The concept of utility has long been a basic underpinning of economic theory. Utility, in general, is the subjective value ascribed to the possession of a good or service or of a particular state of being. Utility is, in essence, someone's preference for something relative to something else. The someone need not be the actual consumer of a service or the person whose state is being assessed.

Utility analysis, as employed in CUA, is based on the work of von Neumann and Morgenstern (1953) (NM) for ranking risky situations. Whenever outcomes cannot be known with certainty, but can be described only in terms of probabilities, then the NM approach is useful. The NM approach has been employed extensively in analyzing gambling, theories of insurance, and wage premiums for risky occupations. In the NM approach, utility values are derived for an individual based on that person's preferences among pairs of gambles. Because health states represent different outcomes with associated probabilities of occurrence (that is, gambles), this method is especially suited to assessing health state utilities.

12.1 Cost-Utility Analysis and Health State Utilities

In socioeconomic evaluation, utilities are employed in the denominator of CUA. In this study type, inputs or costs are measured in economic terms, while the consequences of an intervention are measured in quality-adjusted life years (QALYs). Basically, CUA is an extension of CEA in which years of life are weighted by a factor that incorporates the quality of those life-years. Because of the unique methodology employed and the richness of information that results from CUAs, this form of analysis warrants treatment as a separate study type.

Analysts interested in performing a CUA may be able to obtain utility values for a particular patient group or condition from previously published studies. For example, utility values are available for angina patients (Pliskin et al. 1980), renal failure patients on hemodialysis and continuous peritoneal dialysis (Churchill et al. 1984), laryngectomy patients (McNeil et al. 1981), survivors of neonatal intensive care (Boyle et al. 1983), diabetic patients (Kaplan et al. 1987), and a variety of other conditions (Sackett and Torrance 1978).

12.2 Methods for Assessing Health State Utilities

For those conditions whose health state utilities have not been assessed, the weighting factors can be obtained by a number of methods. The most commonly used methods include the rating scale, the standard gamble, and the time trade-off approaches. Essentially these methods entail asking (usually) to state their preferences when confronted with particular health states. Details of assigning utility values based on these techniques can be obtained in Torrance (1986) and Drummond et al. (1987).

The rating scale method requires presenting respondents with a line anchored on one end by a least desirable health state (0.0) and by a most desirable health state on the other (1.0). Respondents are then provided with detailed descriptions of other health states that would presumably fall between these two extremes. They are asked to represent their preferences about being in these health states by placing them along the line in positions that convey their relative standing to one another and to the end points. The researcher affixes probabilities to each state according to their positions on the scale.

The standard gamble method is directly derived from the NM approach. In this method, respondents are presented with two possible paths or options. The first option is a certainty: the respondent will live in a chronically ill health state (which is described in detail) for a given number of years. The second option involves a gamble. The respondent is faced with two possible outcomes, each associated with a particular probability of occurring. The first outcome is perfect health; the second

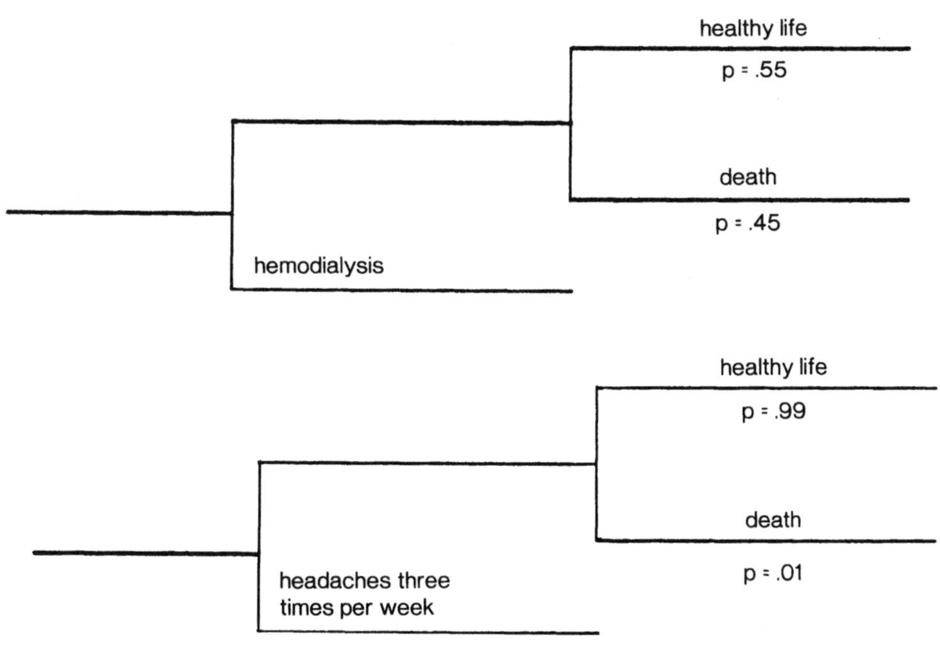

Fig. 12.1. Two possible outcomes of the standard gamble approach to measuring health state utilities

is immediate death. The researcher varies the probabilities that each of these two outcomes will occur until the respondent is equally likely to choose the certain outcome of the chronic health state as he would be to choose the gamble between life or death. Presumably, when confronted with a chronic health state that is extremely onerous, the respondent will choose the certain outcome of that chronic health state only when the probability of living in the healthy state is quite low. On the other hand, when a chronic health state is not very serious, it would be chosen when the probability of dying is very small. Figure 12.1 depicts these two hypothetical situations.

The time trade-off method is a simpler derivation of the standard gamble. In this method, the respondent is confronted with two options. The first option is life in a chronically ill state for a certain length of time. The second option is a healthy life for a shorter period. The researcher varies the time in the healthy state until the respondent is equally likely to choose the healthy state as the ill state.

The utility values that are obtained from these methods can then be combined with measures of the number of life years which are estimated to be associated with interventions to produce the outcome measure quality adjusted life year.

Further Reading

Boyle MH, Torrance GW, Sinclair JC, Horwood SP (1983) Economic evaluation of neonatal intensive care of very-low-birth-weight infants. N Eng J Med 308:1330–1337

Churchill DN, Lemon BC, Torrance GW (1984) A cost-effectiveness analysis of continuous ambulatory peritoneal dialysis and hospital hemodialysis. Med Decis Making 4:489–500

Drummond MF, Stoddart GL, Torrance GW (1987) Methods for the economic evaluation of health care programmes. Oxford Medical, Oxford

Kaplan RM, Hartwell SL, Wilson DK, Wallace JP (1987) Effects of diet and exercise interventions on control and quality of life in non-insulin-dependent diabetes mellitus. J Gen Intern Med 2:220–228

McNeil BJ, Weichselbaum R, Pauker SG (1981) Speech and survival: trade-offs between quality and quantity of life in laryngeal cancer. N Eng J Med 305:982–987

Pliskin JS, Shepard DS, Weinstein MC (1980) Utility functions for life years and health status. Operat Res 28:206–224

Sackett DL, Torrance GW (1978) The utility of different health states as perceived by the general public. J Chronic Dis 31:697–704

Torrance GW (1986) Measurement of health state utilities for economic appraisal. J Health Econ 5:1–30

Von Neumann J, Morgenstern O (1953) Theory of games and economic behavior. Wiley, New York

13 Background on Statistics: Fundamental Concepts

When examining the effect of a certain medication, for example, an antihypertensive, there are two basic options. First, the medication could be given to all hypertensives, that is to the entire *population* of hypertensives. Alternatively, a *sample* of individuals from the population could be chosen and the medication could be given to that sample. The first option is, of course, prohibitively expensive and not feasible. Therefore, the second option is chosen.

The fundamental goal of statistics is to learn about certain important characteristics in a population by looking at only a small sample of the population. *Inferences* could be made about the population based on the data available from the sample. (Hence the name *inferential statistics.)* Statistics provides a particular level of assurance that the correct conclusions are being drawn.

13.1 Measures of Central Tendency and Dispersion

There are several measures of central tendency, or ways of summarizing data from a group of people. The most common is the *mean* or the arithmetic average. The *median* is the value which is the midpoint in the distribution of data. That is, if all the blood pressures for a group of patients were sorted and put in order from highest to lowest, the median would be the value above which half of the group falls and below which the other half of the group falls. The *mode* is the most common value, the one that occurs the most often.

A *normal distribution* has a mean, median, and mode that are equal. Another attribute of a normal distribution is that the individual values fall in a characteristic "bell-shaped curve" around the mean. Figure 13.1 illustrates several normal distributions.

The difference between these distributions is the way in which the individual values are scattered around the mean, or how they are dispersed. There are two primary measures of dispersion: *variance* and *standard deviation.* The variance is computed by finding the difference between each value and the mean, squaring the differences, summing them, and then dividing by the number of cases. The following formula illustrates the concept of variance:

$$\text{Variance} = \frac{\text{sum of (each value} - \text{mean)}^2}{\text{number of subjects}}$$

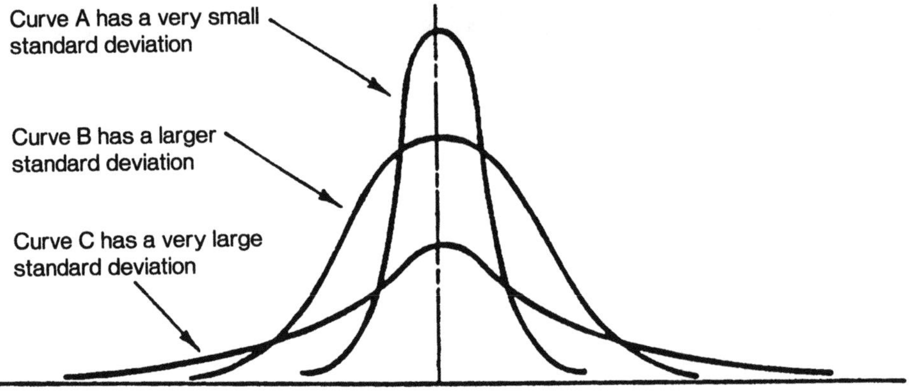

Fig. 13.1. Normal distributions with different standard deviations. (Levin 1981)

The standard deviation is the square root of the variance. Basically, standard deviation and variance are measures of how widely the values are scattered. Curve A is a group of patients who all score very close to the mean and therefore this distribution has a small variance. Curve C represents a group of subjects with a very large variance or standard deviation.

13.2 Hypothesis Testing

When a research study is conducted, the researchers are interested in answering a certain question. For example, they may ask whether this new antihypertensive drug is more effective than placebo at reducing blood pressure. Implicit in this question is a hypothesis:

"The new medication is better than placebo therapy at reducing blood pressure."

However, because it is not possible to prove beyond a shadow of a doubt that this medication is truly better, researchers will test the *null hypothesis:*

"The new medication is *not* more effective than placebo therapy in reducing blood pressure."

The null hypothesis is represented by the Symbol H_0. The research hypothesis is also called the *alternative hypothesis* and is represented by the symbol H_a. If blood pressures in the treatment group are significantly lower than in the placebo group, then the null hypothesis is *rejected,* that is, a *statistically significant difference* between the groups is found.

13.3 Statistical Significance

Before beginning a study, researchers will set a level of significance that is acceptable to them. Generally, this level is set at 0.05. What this means is that the researchers are willing to accept a 5% chance of concluding that there is a difference between the groups when in actuality there is no difference. This level is also called the *alpha* (α) or *P value*. Another way of looking at this is: for any given study, there is a 5% chance of being wrong.

A very important point to make here is that statistical significance is not the same as clinical significance. For example, in the antihypertensive study it is possible that a difference of 1 mmHg between the groups would be significantly different by our statistical standards. (This could happen with very large sample sizes, a topic which will be discussed later.) However, clinically this may mean virtually nothing in terms of reducing the risks of stroke and cardiovascular disease. Thus, the difference is not meaningful from the clinical perspective.

Furthermore, statistical significance, and even clinical significance, does not necessarily imply policy relevance. A certain difference in blood pressure may have clinical significance in that there is a corresponding reduction in the risk for developing hypertensive complications. However, that reduction in risk may translate to a very small proportion of people who are actually affected. For example, it may mean that 0.0001% of individuals will reduce their risk for developing these complications. Given resource expenditure required to result in this reduction of risk, a policymaker might decide that the results of the study do not warrant adoption and use of the medication. This is where a socioeconomic evaluation can be of benefit.

Statistical significance is thus a necessary but insufficient condition for clinical and policy significance. What is generally reported, however, is only the statistical significance of a result. It is up to readers to decide how relevant the results are to their situations and interests.

It was mentioned above that a typical alpha level is 0.05. When researchers set a larger *P* value (e.g., 0.10) they are saying that they are willing to accept a larger probability of being wrong. This is often the case in exploratory studies. When a smaller alpha is set (for example, 0.01 or 0.001), the researchers are saying that they have very strict criteria for judging a significant difference. They want to take fewer chances of saying there is a difference when indeed there is none.

It seems that if researchers wanted to avoid the possibility of concluding that there was a difference when none really existed, they would set extremely small *P* values. However, the less likely we are to make this type of error, the more likely we are to make another type of error. These errors are described next.

13.4 Type I and Type II Error

In reality, there are two possible conditions when comparing two treatment groups: there may be no difference or there may be a difference between the two groups. However, we are not privy to this information and, if we knew it, there would be no reason to perform the study. The only information available to us is the result of the statistical test just performed. In our test there are also two possible conditions: our test may show no difference between the groups or it may show that there is a difference.

When the test shows that there is a significant difference between the groups, but in reality there is *no* difference, then a type I error results. The probability of committing this type of error is under researchers' control when they set the sig-

Table 13.1. Possible outcomes of significance testing

In reality there is:	Our study shows: No difference	Our study shows: Difference
No difference:	Correct decision	Type I error (alpha)
Difference	Type II error (beta)	Correct decision (1-beta or power)

nificance (or alpha) level. This outcome is shown in the upper right-hand quadrant of Table 13.1.

Another type of mistake possible in significance testing is a type II error. This is the probability of saying there is *no* difference between the two groups when in reality there *is* a difference. This is shown in the lower right-hand quadrant of Table 13.1. The less likely we are to commit a type I error, the more likely we are to commit a type II error. The probability of committing a type II error is called beta. Researchers do not directly control this probability as they control the probability of a type I error. Rather, researchers have control over *power,* which is defined as 1-beta.

13.5 Power

Power is the probability of findings a significant difference in our test when there actually is a difference in reality. In other words, it is the probability of making a correct decision when there are statistically significant differences between the groups. This is shown in the lower left-hand quadrant of Table 13.1. In statistics, the goal is to balance power and type I error. We wish to protect ourselves against being too liberal and identifying differences where they do not exist. On the other hand, we wish to find differences that do in fact exist.

To calculate power requires knowledge of three things:

1. Sample size in our groups
2. Expected difference between the groups (also called the size effect)
3. Sample variance

A statistician is usually consulted to perform these calculations. What is important for the reader to recognize is that when a study reports no difference between two treatment groups one possible explanation is that there was insufficient power to detect the differences that were, in fact, present. Very often this error is attributable to an insufficient sample size.

13.6 Sample Size

A technical description of sample size determination is beyond the scope of this chapter; however, the importance of sample size and its influence on our ability to draw conclusions from studies warrants a separate discussion of the issue.

Sample size refers to the number of patients or cases under analysis in a study. The basic question is, how large a sample size is large enough? There is a trade-off between conserving research resources and being able to state without ambiguity that the results of the study are believable.

Sample sizes that are extremely large will enable researchers to detect statistically significant differences when the differences between the groups are very small (that is, the effect size is small). Conversely, if the sample size is too small, then there is a greater probability that true differences will not be detected by the test. This means that power is low.

There are four concepts that are very closely allied with sample size. These are power, variance, significance level, and effect size.

If researchers want their study to have a large degree of *power,* the required sample size increases. In other words, if we want to have greater certainty that we will be able to show statistically significant differences when, in fact, differences exist, it is necessary to have a large sample size. Table 13.2 illustrates this relationship.

As the *variance* in measurements increases, the sample size must increase in order to be able to detect the same level of differences between the groups. (Recall that variance is a measure of the dispersion of actual values around the population mean.) It should make intuitive sense that when there is more variability in the values for individuals in the population from which our sample is drawn, a larger sample size is needed in order to detect differences between the groups. Anything a researcher can do to reduce variability that is not attributable to the treatment will increase power. In other words, if all the variability in an outcome is due to the treatment, our ability to detect significant differences is enhanced. The quest to reduce variance is seen when researchers limit the sample to homogeneous subgroups of the population, such as male hypertensives between the ages of 40 and 50 years with no coexisting morbidity.

Another determinant of sample size is *level of significance.* The more stringently the significance level is set, the larger the sample size required to detect the same level of differences. If we are willing to accept only a 1% chance (alpha = 0.01) of making a type I error (that is, saying there is a difference according to our

Table 13.2. Relationship between power and sample size

Power	Sample size[a]
0.99	232
0.95	168
0.90	138
0.85	119
0.80	106
0.75	95
0.70	85
0.65	77
0.50	57

[a] Sample size required per group to detect a statistically significant difference (alpha = 0.05) between groups which have an expected difference in proportions of 20 percentage points, i.e., 35% in group 1 and 55% in group 2. (Fleiss 1981)

Table 13.3. Relationship between significance level and sample size

Significance level	Sample size[a]
0.01	153
0.02	133
0.05	106
0.10	85
0.20	65

[a] Sample size required per group to detect a statistically significant difference between groups which have an expected difference in proportions of 20 percentage points, i.e., 35% in group 1 and 55% in group 2 at a power level of 0.80 (Fleiss 1981).

test results when in actuality there is none) then we will need a larger sample size than if we set alpha at 0.05 or 0.10. Table 13.3 illustrates this effect.

A final determinant of sample size is the actual difference between the two groups, that is, the *effect size* or the distance between the group means. The larger the difference between two groups the greater the likelihood of detecting that difference and, therefore, the smaller the sample size required.

Table 13.4 illustrates this relationship. If the expected difference between the groups is only 5 percentage points, then 1511 subjects are required to detect a significant difference. In other words, if 35% of group 1 has an improvement in blood pressure and 40% of group 2 shows improvement, then a very large sample size is required to show that this difference is statistically significant. On the other hand, when the effect size is large, for example, when there is a 60 percentage point spread, then only 12 subjects are required per group. The more influence the treatment has on the outcome measure, the smaller the sample size that is required.

Table 13.4. Relationship between effect size and sample size

Effect size		Sample size[a]
Group 1	Group 2	
35%	40%	1511
35%	45%	395
35%	50%	230
35%	55%	106
35%	60%	69
35%	65%	61
35%	70%	45
35%	75%	28
35%	80%	22
35%	85%	18
35%	90%	14
35%	95%	12

[a] Sample size required per group to detect a statistically significant difference (alpha = 0.05) between groups at a power level of 0.80 (Fleiss 1981).

Further Reading

Achen CH (1982) Interpreting and using regression. Sage, Beverly Hills (Sage University paper series on quantitative applications in the social sciences, 07–029)

Anderson S, Auqui A, Hauck WW, et al. (1980) Statistical methods for rates and proportions. Wiley, New York

Carmines EG, Zeller RA (1979) Reliability and validity assessment. Sage, Beverly Hills (Sage University paper series on quantitative applications in the social sciences, 07–017)

Fleiss JL (1981) Statistical methods for rates and proportions, Wiley, New York

Henkel RE (1976) Tests of significance. Sage, Beverly Hills (Sage University paper series on quantitative applications in the social sciences, 07–004)

Huck SW, Cormier WH, Bounds WG (1974) Reading statistics and research. Harper and Row, New York

Iversen GR, Norpoth H (1976) Analysis of variance, Sage, Beverly Hills (Sage University paper series on quantitative applications in the social sciences, 07–001)

Kane EJ (1968) Economic statistics and economics. Harper and Row, New York

Levin RI (1981) Statistics for management. Prentice-Hall, Englewood Cliffs

Lewis-Beck MS (1980) Applied regression: an introduction. Sage, Beverly Hills (Sage University paper series on quantitative applications in the social sciences, 07–022)

Mason RD, Lind DA, Marchal WG (1983) Statistics: an introduction. Harcourt Brace Jovanovich, New York

Neter J, Wasserman W, Kutner MH (1985) Applied linear statistical models. Irwin, Homewood

Stockey E, Zeckhauser R (1978) A primer for policy analysis, Norton, New York

14 Basic Analytical Techniques

This chapter will briefly describe several of the more commonly-used analytic techniques in research reports. This chapter is not meant to serve as a self-contained tutorial on the use of these techniques; however, it should provide the reader with a fundamental understanding of how to interpret these statistical tests.

14.1 Levels of Measurement

Before introducing specific analytical techniques, it is important to understand that there are differences between types of data which depend on how they are measured. The choice of analytical technique is contingent upon the type of data. Essentially there are three different types of data: nominal, ordinal, and interval.

Nominal (also called classificatory or frequency) data are data that simply count the occurrences of a certain characteristic. When information can be classified into categories and there is no specific order to the categories, these are is nominal data. Table 14.1 portrays nominal data.

Table 14.1. Example of nominal data

Marital status	Group A	Group B
Married	30	23
Separated	3	2
Divorced	9	13
Widowed	0	1
Never married	8	1

Ordinal (also called ranked or ordered) data are arrayed in a particular order. This means that the data are ranked with one category being higher or lower than another. Table 14.2 provides an example of data that are ordinal.

Table 14.2. Example of ordinal data

How would you rate your current health status?	
Rating	Number of respondents
Excellent	45
Good	30
Fair	20
Poor	5

Interval (also called score or continuous) data are not only ordered, but the intervals between the data points are constant. Good examples of interval level data are scores from IQ tests, scores on other questionnaire scales, age, and income. Interval level data can be summarized as a mean score. Proportions (i.e., percentages) can be treated as interval level data because the values range from 0 to 100 and the distance between the values is constant.

14.2 Parametric and Nonparametric Tests

There are two broad categories of statistical tests. Parametric tests are performed when it can be assumed that the sample of values in the study was drawn from a normally distributed population (see Chapter 13). This means that the data must be interval level. In addition, the variance in the groups being examined should be equal. This is called "homogeneity of variance." Nonparametric tests are also called distribution-free tests. This means that no assumptions are made about the underlying distribution of data nor about the variances of the groups.

In general, parametric tests have greater *power,* that is, they are able to point out statistically significant differences when they truly exist. Some researchers feel that even when the two basic assumptions for parametric tests do not hold true, it is still better to use parametric tests. Nonparametric tests should be used with extremely small sample sizes (say, less than 25) and when the underlying populations are extremely "nonnormal", that is, when the distribution is extremely skewed.

The only nonparametric test to be discussed here is the chi-square test; however, Table 14.3 provides a comparison of parametric and other nonparametric tests.

Table 14.3. Analogous parametric and nonparametric tests. (Adapted from Huck et al. 1974)

Parametric	Nonparametric
Pearson product moment correlation coefficient (r)	Spearman rank-order correlation coefficient (rho)
t-Test	Sign test Mann-Whitney U test
One-way ANOVA	Kruskal Wallis one-way ANOVA or ranks
(No analogous test)	Chi-square test

14.3 Commonly Used Statistical Techniques

14.3.1 t-Test

The simplest comparison between two groups aimed at detecting statistically significant differences is the t-test. t-tests are used under the following conditions: a) the outcome scores are reported as a mean (or average), and thus the data are interval level; b) it is assumed that the subjects were randomly drawn from a larger population; and c) it is assumed that the population has a normal distribution and the variance is unknown.

If the difference between the means of the two groups is great enough, then the *t*-test will be significant. When researchers report the results of the *t*-test, they usually report the calculated value and a *p*-value. The calculated value is the result of computing the *t*-test formula. (Readers should consult a statistics textbook to obtain this formula and the others mentioned later.) The researcher then looks up this value in a statistical table and obtains the *p*-value.

As a general rule of thumb, calculated *t*-values greater than approximately 2 are significant at an alpha level of 0.05 for larger sample sizes (say, over 100). In a study that is testing the effect of a certain treatment, this indicates that the group means were far enough apart to conclude that the intervention really did have an effect on the group which received the treatment. Often the researcher will report a specific *t*-value and *p*-value in the following manner:

$t = 3.20^*$ $\quad ^*p < 0.01$

This means that the calculated value that resulted from computing the *t*-test formula was 3.20. When the researcher looked this up in the table, the associated *p*-value was smaller than 0.01.

t-tests can be one-tailed or two-tailed tests. (To understand what is meant by the "tail," refer to Fig. 13.1 in the previous chapter. The tail is that portion of the distribution curve that approaches the horizontal axis.) For example, a two-tailed test is performed when the researcher is not certain whether drug A will be better or worse than drug B. A one-tailed test is performed when the researcher has reason to believe that drug A is better than (or worse than) drug B. The important thing to recall about one- and two-tailed tests is that alpha levels do not mean the same thing in these two tests. If the researcher set the alpha at 0.05 in a two-tailed test, the alpha is actually divided by 2. As a result, a two-tailed test is more stringent: significant differences are less likely when using a two-tailed test than when using a one-tailed test.

The reader may encounter the *z*-test in certain studies. This is interpreted in a similar fashion to *t*-tests. It is applicable to testing proportions as well as means and is used when the population variances are known.

14.3.2 Analysis of Variance

When researchers want to compare the mean scores for more than two groups, it would be possible to use *t*-tests to make pair-wise comparisons, that is, for three groups (A, B, and C) they would compare A with B, A with C, and B with C. This would require conducting three separate *t*-tests. Not only is this inconvenient, but a statistical problem arises as well. Say every *t*-test is performed with an alpha level of 0.05. When two tests are performed, the *experiment-wise alpha* is not 0.05, but 0.10. When three tests are performed, the experiment-wise alpha increases to 0.15. This means that the chance of a type I error is now 0.15, or there is a 15% chance of saying that a difference exists when in reality there is no difference.

To avoid this problem, analysis of variance (ANOVA) can be used. ANOVA is an extention of the *t*-test. (When ANOVA is used to compare two groups, the results will be identical to those of a *t*-test.) ANOVA can be used for comparing the group means of three or more groups; thus the data must again be interval level. All the assumptions that apply to the *t*-test also apply to ANOVA: the variances are equal, the populations are normally distributed, and the samples are independent and randomly selected.

Because ANOVA originated in agricultural research, the different groups are often called *treatments* rather than groups. The variable used to group the patients is called the *independent variable* or the *factor*. For example, in a comparison of three different medication dosages (50, 100, and 150 mg) and a placebo, the independent variable is medication, and it has four *levels* or categories into which patients are grouped.

The results of an ANOVA are often presented in a summary table such as the one displayed in Table 14.4.

Table 14.4. Sample ANOVA summary table

Source of variation	Degrees of freedom	Sum of squares	Mean square	F
Between groups (also called treatment or factor)	$k-1$	SSB	$\frac{\text{SSB}}{k-1}$	$\frac{\text{SST}/(k-1)}{\text{SSE}/(N-k)}$
Within groups (also called error)	$N-k$	SSE	$\frac{\text{SSE}}{N-k}$	
Total		SST		

k, number of groups; N, total number of subjects; SSB, sums of squares between the groups; this is the difference between the groups that is attributable to the treatment; SSE, sums of squares error; this is the difference that is attributable to random error; SST, sums of square total; this is the total difference between the groups, or the summation of SSB and SSE

The test statistic for ANOVA is the *F*-test. This is based on the *F* distribution, which is positively skewed and always positive; that is, it ranges from zero to infinity. There are differently shaped *F* distributions depending on the degrees of freedom (which are based on the sample size and the number of groups). The *F* statistic is computed using the results displayed in the summary table and is interpreted as a critical value in the same manner as the *t* statistic.

If an ANOVA is conducted on three or more groups and the *F* statistic is significant, then the null hypothesis of equal group means can be rejected. However, there is still uncertainty regarding which groups differ from the others, and where the differences lie. In a comparison of three groups (A, B, and C), there are four possible outcomes:

A ≠ B, A ≠ C, B = C (the mean of group A differs from B and C, but the means of groups B and C are not significantly different)

B ≠ A, B ≠ C, A = C (the mean of group B differs from A and C, but the means of groups A and C are not different)

C ≠ A, C ≠ B, A = B (the mean of group C differs from A and B, but the means of groups A and B are not different)

A ≠ B, B ≠ C, A ≠ C (all three groups differ from one another).

When 4 groups are compared, there are 14 possible outcomes. When 5 groups are compared, there are 56 possible outcomes. To discern which groups are different from one another, researchers often perform comparisons called *post hoc techniques*. There are several post hoc comparison techniques available which range from conservative to liberal tests. A liberal test will tend to find statistically significant differences when the group means are rather close together, while a conservative test will not find significant differences until the group means are quite far apart. The most commonly used technique is also the most conservative and is called the *Scheffé test*.

The ANOVA described above is called a *one-way ANOVA*. This is because there is only one independent variable, that is, there is only one variable or dimension along which subjects are placed into groups. ANOVA can accommodate two or more independent variables with two or more levels in each. When there are two independent variables, it is called a *two-way ANOVA;* three independent variables yield a *three-way ANOVA*. When two or more independent variables are examined, this is also termed *factorial ANOVA*. A one-way ANOVA examines one *effect* or dimension along which the groups can differ. Whenever a factorial ANOVA is performed, there is an increase in the number of effects that can be observed. For example, say one factor is medication dosage with four levels (50, 100, and 150 mg, and placebo) and the other factor is health care setting with two levels (inpatient and outpatient). This is termed a 4 × 2 factorial ANOVA (referring to the number of levels in each factor). There are three possible effects that can be examined in this analysis: the main effect for medication dosage, the main effect for health care setting, and the interaction effect between medication and health care setting. *Interaction* refers to the joint effect of medication and health care setting operating in unison. What this means is that the effect of the medication dosage may vary according to the health care setting in which the medication is delivered. This is an important concept because it takes into account the fact that the presence of one variable alone may have a different effect on the dependent variable of interest than that variable in the presence of another variable.

14.3.3 Chi-square Test

When data are nominal or ordinal level (that is, the data are categorical or frequency), then the chi-square test is appropriate. The chi-square test is the most commonly used nonparametric test. It is based on the chi-square distribution which is positively skewed and always positive. Like the *F* distribution, there are numerous chi-square distributions according to the degrees of freedom, but as the degrees of freedom become large enough the chi-square distribution tends to become symmetrical, like a normal distribution.

The chi-square test can be used to test *goodness-of-fit,* that is, how well the observed frequencies in the categories match the expected frequencies. Another term for this is the single-sample chi-square test. What we are trying to discover in conducting a goodness-of-fit test is whether the number of subjects that are observed to fall into these categories matches the number we would expect to fall into the categories by chance. For example, say there are four floors in the hospital with an equal number of beds on each. For the sake of simplicity, assume that patients are assigned to the floors in a random way, so that we would not expect one floor to have sicker patients than any other floor. The hospital director is interested in finding out if hospital-acquired infection rates are occurring in a pattern that could be explained by chance. The data collected from the hospital records are displayed in Table 14.5.

Table 14.5. Data used in chi-square goodness of fit test

Floor	Expected	Observed
1	10	12
2	10	3
3	10	16
4	10	9

After performing the calculations, the director ended up with a chi-square value of 9.0. At an alpha level of 0.05 this is statistically significant and the director can reject the null hypothesis. The conclusion is that the differences observed could not have occurred simply by chance. The calculations become a little more complex when the expected cell frequencies are not the same, but the interpretation of the statistical results does not change.

Another frequently used application of the chi-square test is *contingency table analysis,* also called the independent samples chi-square test. Where the goodness-of-fit test examines only one variable or level of categorization, contingency table analysis cross-classifies variables. An example of a contingency table is presented in Table 14.6.

Table 14.6. Example of a contingency table

	Group assignment		
Gender	Control group	Experimental group	Total
Male	48	52	100
Female	51	49	100
Total	100	100	200

Again, this chi-square test is based on comparing the observed frequencies in the cells with the expected frequencies and we are interested in determining whether the expected frequencies could have occurred by chance. The null hypothesis for a contingency table analysis states that the two factors which are examined are unrelated to one another. In the contingency table above, the chi-square statistic is very small and therefore is not significant. We can conclude that the differences in the observed frequencies could indeed have occurred by chance and that gender is not related to group assignment.

One word of caution: when cell sizes are small, say fewer than five, the chi-square test loses reliability. The chi-square statistic will be too large (that is to say, too liberal) and even small differences may be considered statistically significant. In such situations, a correction factor called Yates correction should be reported or adjacent cells should be combined to form larger cell sizes.

14.3.4 Correlation Analysis

Correlation analysis is used to examine the strength of the relationship between two variables. When the variables are ordinal or nominal (categorical), then Spearman's rank order correlation coefficient (rho) is used. When the variables are measured at the interval (continuous) level, then the Pearson product moment correlation *(r)* is used. This is the most commonly utilized form of correlation analysis.

The correlation coefficient is termed r. The relationship between two variables can range from a high positive correlation ($r = +1.0$) to no correlation ($r = 0$) to a high negative correlation ($r = -1.0$). When variables are positively correlated, their relationship is termed *direct;* when they are negatively correlated, their relationship is *inverse.*

The *coefficient of determination* is termed r^2 and results from squaring the correlation coefficient *(r)*. It describes the proportion of variation in one variable that is explained or accounted for by another variable. For example, an r^2 value of 0.67 means that variable *A* explains 67% of the variability in variable *B*. Thus, 33% of the variation in values of variable *B* are explained by other factors.

It is possible to test the significance of a correlation coefficient. The null hypothesis is that the correlation coefficient is actually zero, that is, the two variables are not related to one another. The reader should be warned, however, that a statistically significant correlation coefficient does not indicate that the correlation between the two variables is strong. This is a judgment which is solely based on the correlation coefficient. In other words, a correlation coefficient that is not statistically significant indicates that the relationship between two variables is negligible. But a statistically significant coefficient does not indicate a strong relationship. In addition, the reader should not make the mistake of confusing correlation with causality. A strong correlation only indicates that a relationship exists, it does not say anything about which variable caused the other. Indeed, it is possible that a third variable may be the true cause of one or the other or both.

One way of reporting correlation coefficients is in a correlation matrix. This is a cross-classification of variables and their correlation coefficients. Table 14.7 is an illustration of a correlation matrix.

First, note that the upper right half of the matrix is a mirror image of the lower left half. Many reports present correlation matrices with only one half or the other. Second, all the diagonal cells contain 1.00, which indicates that each variable is perfectly correlated with itself. Third, all the coefficients are statistically significant, although correlations in the range of 0.20 to 0.40 would be considered low to moderate in strength.

Table 14.7. Correlation matrix of compliance measures

Compliance measures	Pill count	Lithium level	Appointment keeping
Pill count	1.00	0.49[b]	0.42[b]
Lithium level	0.49[b]	1.00	0.21[a]
Appointment keeping	0.42[b]	0.21[a]	1.00

[a] Significant at 0.05
[b] Significant at 0.01

14.3.5 Ordinary Least Squares Regression

Ordinary least squares (OLS) regression, also called *linear regression,* is a statistical method which measures the relationship between two or more variables. When there are only two variables it is termed simple regression. When several variables (independent variables) are used to explain another variable (the dependent variable), it is termed *multiple regression.*

Regression is used under the following conditions:

1. There is one dependent variable which will be explained using at least one independent variable.
2. All variables are measured at the interval (continuous) level.
3. The regression assumptions are met. (These will be mentioned later. However, a discussion of these assumptions is beyond the scope of this chapter.)

The basic principle behind regression is *least squares analysis.* One way to examine the relationship between two variables is to draw a *scatterplot* or a *scatter diagram* of them. Figure 14.1 is an example of a scatterplot.

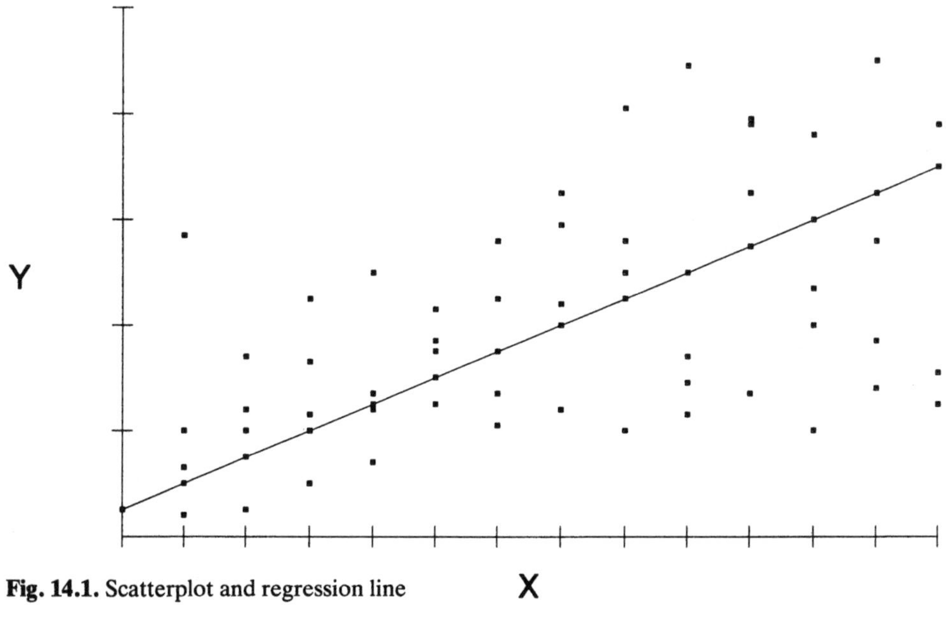

Fig. 14.1. Scatterplot and regression line

X is the predictor variable and Y is the value of the variable which is predicted by X. Each variable of interest is placed on its own axis, and the intersecting data points are plotted. It is possible to draw straight lines through these points that would tend to define the "average" of all the points. There is a potentially very large number of lines that can be fitted through the scatter of observations and some lines will represent the data better than others. However, through least squares analysis this line could be placed much more accurately. Least squares analysis looks at each data point in a scatterplot in terms of how far the point lies from the imaginary line that would best represent the relationship between X and Y. The distances are described as *deviations* or *errors*. Least squares regression then squares all these deviations and sums them for many potential lines. The line that has the smallest value for these *sums of squares* is the regression line. Thus linear regression analysis is based on the search and identification of such a line which minimizes the sum of squared deviations of individual data points from the corresponding point on the fitted line.[1]

In multiple regression, X represents the independent variables and Y represents the dependent variable. The regression equation with two independent variables is written as:

$$Y = a + b_1 X_1 + b_2 X_2$$

The term *"a"* equals the *y* intercept, which is where the regression line crosses the upright axis in a scatter diagram. The intercept is interpreted as the value of Y when all the Xs are equal to zero. The term *"b"* is called the slope of the regression line. It refers to how steeply the regression rises or falls. A large positive number indicates a steep slope going upward, while a small negative number indicates a shallow slope going downward. The slope is also called the regression coefficient, or beta. The betas are interpreted as the change in the dependent variable *(Y)* that accompanies a one-point increase in the independent variable *(X)*. The X terms are independent variables. For each combination of X terms there will be a corresponding Y value. These are the data points on the scatterplot.[2] In linear regression there can be multiple independent variables, but only one dependent variable.

The *standard error of the estimate* is a measure of how far the data points are scattered away from the regression line. In other words, it measures the variability of the observed values of Y from the predicted values of Y. When the standard error of the estimate is small, this means that the regression line fits the data quite closely. When it is large, there is considerable error in the estimation of Y, that is, the deviations from the line of best fit are large.

---

[1] Linear regression is based on several assumptions about the observations and their errors, or deviations from the line of best fit. The reader is encouraged to consult a statistical text for a detailed explanation of these assumptions.

[2] Of course, when there are two independent variables the scatterplot becomes considerably more complex as it must take on three dimensions. As more independent variables are added, our theoretical scatterplot would become more and more complex with added dimensions.

When reading a report of a regression analysis, there are several common terms and concepts used. The regression equation may be displayed. This is an example of a regression equation:

$$Y = 5.43 + 2.67\,X_1 - 4.77\,X_2 - 1.54\,X_3$$

For example, the beta coefficient of -1.54 means that for every one point increase in X_3 there is a 1.54-point decline in Y. The intercept is 5.43, which indicates that when all the independent variables are equal to zero the dependent variable has a value of 5.43. (The intercept is generally of limited informational value to the researcher.)

Each coefficient will have a significance value associated with it. The null hypothesis being tested is that the coefficient is not significantly different from zero. If the null hypothesis were true, then that independent variable is not a significant *predictor* of the dependent variable, that is, that X variable does not explain the variation observed in Y.

There are several ways to interpret the equation itself. First we can examine the significance of the equation. Each regression equation will have an associated F-test. This is interpreted exactly as an F-test in an ANOVA. It tests the null hypothesis that the combination of Xs in this equation are not important predictors of Y, that is, they do not explain the variability observed in Y.

Another measure used to interpret the regression equation is the coefficient of multiple determination (R^2). This value tells us what portion of the total variability in Y is explained by all the Xs present in the equation. R^2 can range from 0 to 1.00. 0 indicates that the independent variables explain very little of the variation in Y. An R^2 value of, say 0.57 indicates that the combination of independent variables explains 57% of the variability in Y. An R^2 of 1.00 is perfect; all the variability in Y is explained by this set of Xs. (This rarely occurs.)

Stepwise regression is a type of regression technique in which each independent variable is entered into the equation separately according to its strength as a predictor of Y. Stronger predictors are entered first and weaker ones last. The choice of which variables enter first or later is determined by the statistical strength of the relationship between the independent and the dependent variable. A variation of this is *hierarchical regression* in which groups of independent variables are defined by the researcher as being theoretically more or less important, rather than relying upon the statistical program to determine the order of entry. These groups of variables are then entered into the analysis, one by one.

Glossary

activities of daily living (ADL). Those behaviors that are fundamental to independent living, such as feeding oneself, dressing, bathing, ambulating.

alpha. The level of significance that is specified prior to conducting a statistical test; the probability of a type I error.

alternative hypothesis. A statement about the value of a parameter in the population which claims there *is* a significant effect; this is accepted if the null hypothesis is rejected; also called the research hypothesis, H_a.

analysis of variance (ANOVA). A statistical technique that compares groups in terms of their mean scores; similar to the *t*-test but applicable to more than two groups at a time.

analysis of covariance (ANCOVA). A method that compares the mean scores of two groups after adjusting these means by some other "covariate" or variable that is expected to influence these mean scores.

base case. A condition in a sensitivity analysis, when all variables are assigned their most likely value; the condition against which sensitivity analyses are compared; best estimate.

Bayes' theorem. A formula that allows us to revise probabilities (called posterior probabilities) based on limited information and to change those probabilities as more information is gathered.

benefit. The outcome of using a product or service; output; the term "consequences" may be preferred; the outcome measure in a cost-benefit analysis.

benefit-cost ratio. Commonly used to describe the conclusion of a cost-benefit study. It is the ratio of the present value of benefits to the present value of costs. Given that the classification of some entities as costs or negative benefits, and benefits or negative costs, is ambiguous, the ratio can be a misleading indicator of efficiency. It is better to use the difference between the net present values rather than their ratios.

best estimate. See base case.

beta. In linear regression, the regression coefficient; the slope of the regression line; the change in the dependent variable that accompanies a one-point increase in the independent variable. Also the probability of committing a type II error.

between groups. In analysis of variance, that portion of the variance which is attributable to differences between subjects in different groups; also called between column variance.

bimodal. Having two modes.

blind. A condition in clinical trials when patients are unaware of their assignment to the control or the experimental group; controls for placebo effect.

capital. Viewed variously as a physical stock of assets (buildings, land, plant, equipment, etc.), as a stock of financial assets (government bills, equities, bank balances, etc.), or as the present value of the net value (or netwoth) of a stream of services over time that a particular asset or program may yield.

capital cost. The *cost* of acquiring, owning or using an item of capital equipment net of depreciation.

census. Obtaining information on every element in the population; the opposite of sampling.

charge. The market price associated with a product or service; does not necessarily reflect the economic or opportunity cost.

chi-square. A test of statistical significance for frequency data: also used to test hypotheses regarding variance and goodness-of-fit.

chi-square distribution. A distribution that is positively skewed when applied to small samples, but achieves a nearly normal distribution for larger sample sizes.

coefficient alpha. A measure of the internal consistency or reliability of a scale.

coefficient of determination. The correlation coefficient squared (r^2); the proportion of variance in one variable explained by another variable.

coefficient of multiple determination. In linear regression, R^2; the proportion of the total variability in the dependent variable *(Y)* explained by all the independent variables (*X*s) in a linear regression equation.

comorbidity. A coexisting illness or disease.

confidence interval. A range based on sample estimates that should contain the population parameter with a specified probability, e.g., 95% or 99%; a 95% confidence interval based on sample data indicates that there is probability of 0.95 that the interval includes the population mean.

consequence. The outcome of using a product or service; output; can be measured in economic or other units; see benefit.

constraints. The limits (budgetary, resource, political, etc.) on what it is possible to accomplish. Careful examination of imagined constraints often results in their being seen to be moveable, though usually at some cost.

contingency table. A table that has rows that correspond to levels of one categorical variable and columns that correspond to the levels of another categorical variable; the cells of the table show the frequency of cases that occur in each variable combination; used to assess whether the variables are related to one another; employs the chi-square test.

continuous data. Interval level data; the difference between each value is known and constant, e.g., age.

control group. A characteristic of experimental studies; a group of subjects who are observed but who receive no treatment; provides the researcher with a baseline against which to measure the effect of the treatment.

correlation. The interrelationship or strength of association between variables.

correlation analysis. Statistical techniques that detect the relationship between two variables; the most commonly used technique is Pearson's product moment correlation *(r)*.

correlation coefficient. The statistic that measures the interrelationship between two variables; ranges from 0 (no relationship) to 1 (perfect relationship); *r*.

correlation matrix. Cross-classification of variables and their correlations.

cost-benefit analysis. A form of socioeconomic analysis in which both costs and consequences are expressed in monetary values.

cost-effectiveness analysis. A form of socioeconomic evaluation in which costs are measured in economic terms and at least some consequences are measured in their natural units such as lives saved or years of life saved.

cost-minimization analysis. A form of socioeconomic evaluation that is appropriate when two or more alternatives have equivalent effectiveness and only their costs must be compared: analysis identifies the least costly alternative.

cost-of-illness study. A form of economic evaluation that estimates the economic impact of a disease.

cost-utility analysis. A form of socioeconomic evaluation that measures costs in monetary terms but measures consequences in terms of their quality or utility.

costs. The best alternative use value of the economic inputs that are required to achieve a certain output.

criterion. See dependent variable.

data. Observations on variables of interest.

decision analysis. A predictive technique that is used to analyze the decision-making process and to measure uncertainty; an analytical tool that formally depicts the decision-making process in an attempt to describe the most favorable course of action.

decision tree. A graphic display of possible decisions and outcomes, along with estimated probabilities of each chance event and the utility associated with each outcome.

degrees of freedom. The number of values that can be chosen freely; the number of degrees of freedom in a statistical test equals the number of subjects (the sample size) minus the number of groups.

dependent variable. The variable that is being predicted or estimated; the variable that is affected by the independent variable; denoted by *Y* in multiple regression equations; also called the criterion.

descriptive statistics. Statistics that describe the sample that is being measured; methods of portraying the data collected on a specific group of subjects; there is no attempt at drawing inferences for a larger population.

dichotomous data. Data having one of two possible values, usually coded 0 and 1.

direct costs. Changes in resource use attributable to the intervention being studied; includes both medical and nonmedical resources.

direct relationship. A relationship between two variables: as one increases in value the other increases in value also.

discount factor. See discounting for general description. The discount factor for year t is given by $1/(1 + r)^t$ where r is the annual discount rate. Thus, if $r = 0.1$, the discount factor for $t = 1$ is 0.909 and for $t = 5$ it is 0.620.

discounting. A procedure for reducing flows of cost or benefits occurring at different dates into common measure called the present value by use of an appropriate discount rate. Thus, with an annual discount rate r (expressed as a decimal fraction) the present value (PV) of a cost (C) in 1 year's time is $PV = C/(1 + r)$.

discount rate. The rate of interest used to calculate a present value.

disease costing. A procedure for assigning the expenditures of a health system or part thereof to the particular disease for which care is provided. See cost of illness.

discrete data. Nominal or interval level data; data that are categorical, mutually exclusive, and may or may not be ranked, e.g., marital status or socioeconomic status.

double-blind. A condition in clinical trials when both patient and physician (or researcher) are unaware of the patient's assignment to the control or the experimental group; employed to counteract the placebo effect in patients and to minimize researcher bias in interpreting the results of the experiment.

dummy variable. A variable that is coded 0 or 1; used to transform a continuous level variable or one with multiple categories into a variable that can be analyzed using multiple regression.

economic appraisal. See cost-benefit analysis, cost-effectiveness analysis, cost-utility analysis and financial appraisal.

effect size. The difference between group means; the difference between two groups that may be attributable to a treatment.

effectiveness. The extent to which the output of a product, service, or program meets its objectives as assessed under *normal* operating conditions.

efficiency. In a restrictive sense defined either as minimizing the opportunity cost of attaining a given output or as maximizing the output for a given opportunity cost. The general term used by economists is known as "Pareto-efficiency". This is an allocation of resources such that it is not possible to reallocate them without imposing uncompensated losses on some individual. A variant is "potential Pareto-efficiency", where it is not possible to reallocate resources without imposing uncompensated losses on someone. It is common to see the notion of efficiency expressed at three different levels: technical efficiency, where more inputs are not used than are technically necessary to attain a given output; cost-efficiency, or cost-effectiveness, where a given output is produced using the least-cost technically efficient combination of inputs (or, conversely, output is maximized for a given level of cost); Pareto-efficiency, where output is not only technically and cost efficient but is also set at an efficient rate such that a diminution or increase would impose uncompensated losses on some individual.

epidemiology. The study of the distribution of diseases within a group of individuals; aims at describing the common characteristics among those affected by the disease.

experimental study. A study in which subjects are randomly assigned to groups, an intervention is introduced, and the intervention's effect on the subjects is measured; ambiguity regarding cause and effect is minimized in this type of study.

external validity. The extent to which the results obtained from a study can be generalized to other groups.

F distribution. A positively skewed distribution that is always positive, ranging from zero to infinity; used in the *F*-test for analysis of variance; there are a family of *F*-distributions based on the degrees of freedom in the test.

financial appraisal. A procedure for assessing options that is similar to cost-benefit analysis except that only the financial costs and benefits to an organization are considered, rather than social costs and benefits. Also called budgetary analysis.

F test. A test of statistical significance that tests whether the amount of varibility of one group is different from the variability in another group; based on the *F*-distribution; used in analysis of variance (where more than two groups are being compared).

factor. See independent variable.

factorial design. A research design that has two or more independent variables (or factors), the effects of which are measured separately and in combination, that is, the test examines the effect of variable *A* on *Y*, the effect of variable *B* on *Y*, and the combined effects of variables *A* and *B* (in unison) on *Y*.

false positive. A case that is labeled as having disease, but which in reality is healthy.

fixed cost. Costs that remain constant across the entire range of service volumes.

frequency data. Data organized to show the frequency with which subjects fall into predefined categories or groups.

frequency distribution. A method of arranging data into categories based on the frequency with which each value occurs.

goodness-of-fit test. Used to determine how well an observed set of data match an expected set of data; uses the chi-square test.

Hawthorne effect. A change in subjects' behavior resulting from their knowledge that they are being observed: a confounder that reduces the validity of research results.

hierarchical regression. In linear regression, groups of independent variables are entered into the equation in an order determined by the researcher, usually based on a theoretical assumption of the variables' relative importance as predictors.

histogram. A graph of a frequency distribution using bars whose height represents the number of cases in each category or grouping; also called a bar chart.

human capital approach. A method of valuing indirect cost based on the expected economic productivity of the individual.

hypothesis. A statement about the value of a population parameter.

incidence. The rate of development of a disease in a group over a period of time; the number of persons developing a disease divided by the number of persons at risk per unit of time; the number of *new* cases discovered in a time period; the development of disease.

independent variable. The variable whose value is known; a variable that predicts or has an effect on the dependent variable; denoted by X in multiple regression equations; also called a factor.

indirect costs. Monetary value of the negative changes in the productivity of a patient that result from the intervention.

indirect (or inverse) relationship. A relationship between two variables: as one increases in value, the other decreases in value.

inferential statistics. Analytical methods that use data obtained from a sample to characterize a larger population.

intangible costs. Costs that are not quantifiable in monetary terms.

interaction. The joint effect of two or more independent variables operating in unison on a dependent variable.

internal consistency. A form of estimating the reliability of a scale by computing the correlation between all possible halves of a scale; produces a score called coefficient alpha; contrast with split-half reliability.

internal validity. The extent to which there is no systematic or nonrandom error in the data; the extent to which the results of a study are accurate for the group of patients included in the study; contrast with external validity.

interval. Data that are continuous; the difference between each value is known and constant, e.g., age.

inverse relationship. See indirect relationship.

league table. A table that arrays various medical interventions according to the estimated cost per quality-adjusted life year gained; used for cost-utility analysis.

level. In ANOVA, the categories into which patients are grouped within the independent variable.

life-year. An output measure used in socioeconomic evaluations; computed as the number of affected individuals multiplied by the number of years each person is expected to live.

linear regression. See ordinary least squares regression.

logistic regression. A regression technique appropriate for a dichotomous dependent variable; based on the logistic function (an *s*-shaped distribution); often used to estimate the probability of developing disease.

marginal analysis. Analytical technique that examines the incremental effects of increasing or decreasing inputs.

marginal benefit. The additional incremental benefit that is obtained as a result of additional investment or activity.

marginal cost. The additional incremental investment in resources to obtain additional benefit.

matching. A procedure in which the subjects of one group are individually selected to have identical values on certain key variables to the subjects of another group; these variables are thought to affect the outcome of interest.

mean. The arithmetic average; a measure of central tendency.

median. The exact midpoint of a distribution of data that is ordered from high to low; a measure of central tendency.

medical cost. The direct medical resource inputs associated with a product or service.

mode. The value that occurs most often in a series of data; a measure of central tendency.

modeling. An analytical technique used to simulate processes that occur through time; often used to explain the impact of numerous independent variables on one or more dependent variables; used when experimental techniques are not feasible.

morbidity. Illness or disease, standardised.

mortality. Death, standardised.

multicollinearity. The condition when independent variables in a multiple regression equation are highly correlated with one another; leads to instability of the regression coefficients.

multiple regression. See ordinary least squares regression.

multivariate. Pertaining to many variables.

natural experiment. A quasi-experiment in which an intervention occurs naturally in one group or area and its effect is measured and compared with a group or area not exposed to the intervention.

node. The point on a decision tree where branching occurs; circular symbols on the tree diagram designate chance nodes; square symbols on the tree diagram designate choice (or decision) nodes.

nominal. Data that are categorical, mutually exclusive, and not ranked, e.g., marital status.

nonmedical cost. The direct resource inputs from outside the medical sector associated with a product or service, e.g., transportation to and from medical services, child care, social services.

nonparametric tests. Statistical tests that make no assumptions about the underlying nature of the distribution of the population; appropriate tests for very small sample size (less than 25); tests used when variables are measured on the nominal (categorical) or ordinal (ranked) scale; also called distribution-free statistics; generally not as robust as analogous parametric statistics, that is, these tests are less likely to detect significant differences when they do exist.

normal distribution. A unimodal, bell-shaped, symmetrical distribution whose mean, median, and mode are equal to the same value.

null hypothesis. A statement about the value of a parameter in the population that claims that there is *no* difference or no significant effect; H_0.

objectives. The aims or end-states that are sought in health systems or parts of systems. They may be cast in rather general forms such as "to maximise utility" or more specifically in terms of directly measurable achievement (e.g., number of patients successfully discharged). Useful statements of objectives are normally cast in terms of outputs to be achieved or net benefits to be maximised.

observational study. A study that observes characteristics of subjects without intervening or introducing a treatment.

one-way ANOVA. An ANOVA that compares groups on the basis of one independent variable; see analysis of variance.

one-tailed hypothesis. A research (or alternative) hypothesis that states the expected direction of the difference between two groups; a hypothesis that tests whether one group is greater than or less than another group.

opportunity cost. The true cost of service or product A is the value of the alternative services or products that are forgone as a result of the investment in A; those resources devoted to the production of a certain service or product are not available for investment in other services or products.

option appraisal. The use of cost-benefit analysis and related techniques to select between alternatives and assess the desirability of one relative to another.

ordinal. Data that are categorical, mutually exclusive, and ranked, that is, one category is higher than another, e.g., socioeconomic status.

ordinary least squares regression. A statistical technique that uses multiple independent variables to predict one dependent variable; a multiple regression technique based on minimizing the sum of the squared differences between the observations and the regression line (or between the observed values of the dependent variable and the predicted values); a regression technique appropriate for a continuous dependent variable.

output. The effects produced by production. Changes in health status are the ultimate output of health services. However, sometimes more proximate throughput measures are used such as "patients discharged". In general, the use of inputs as measures of output is not recommended since the practice begs the question as to the nature and amount of output that the inputs may generate, particularly at the margin.

parameter. A measurable characteristic of a population; contrast with statistic.

parametric tests. Statistical tests that make certain important assumptions: (a) the sample on which the statistics are applied was randomly selected from the population, (b) the values in the population have homogeneous variances, and (c) the values have a normal distribution in the population; the most commonly used class of statistics.

pathway of clinical management. Descriptions or models that describe the diagnostic and treatment process, including expected patterns of resource utilization, and possible outcomes after interventions.

Pearson correlation coefficient. A statistic that measures the interrelationship between two interval-level variables; ranges from 0 (no relationship) to +1 or −1 (perfect positive or negative relationship); symbolized by r.

perspective. The viewpoint from which the analysis is conducted.

placebo. A sham treatment; used in clinical trials to control for the patient' s and experimenter's expectations of improving after the administration of treatment.

population. All subjects in a particular group, e.g., the population of the United States, all 1st-year medical students, or all patients with a particular disease. This is the entire group about which inferences are made in statistical analysis.

positive value of time preference. The principle on which discounting is based; holds that costs and benefits that occur in the present have greater value than those that occur in the future.

post hoc comparison. After an ANOVA test has led to a rejection of the null hypothesis, these comparisons are performed to discern where the group differences lie, that is, which specific groups differ from one another; post hoc technique.

power. The probability of rejecting the null hypothesis when it is false; the ability of a statistical test to find significant differences between groups.

present value. See discounting.

pre-test post-test. A one group quasi-experimental design that entails measuring a group of subjects prior to a treatment, introducing a treatment, and then comparing the response to treatment to the pretreatment scores.

prevalence. The number of persons with a disease divided by the number of persons in the total group at any one point in time; the total cases at one point in time; the extent of disease.

primary data. Data that have not been analyzed.

probability. The chance or likelihood that an event will occur; defined as the number of outcomes where the event occurs divided by the total number of outcomes.

probit regression. A regression technique appropriate for a dichotomous dependent variable; based on the cumulative normal probability function; results in coefficients that can be interpreted only in light of the values of other dependent variables.

production function. A description of the resources required to produce a service or product, how the resources are combined, and what possible outcomes might be expected.

prospective. A study in which data are collected during the study; a study that follows a group of patients through time with periodic evaluations.

QUALY. See *quality adjusted life year.*

quality adjusted life year (QALY). Life years weighted by a utility value that measures the relative quality of life experienced.

quality of life. The social, physiological, mental, intellectual, and general well-being of individuals. An index of the quality of a year of life, usually measured by a utility number and embodying the value judgments of selected judges. (QALY = quality − adjusted life − year).

quasi-experiment. A study in which an intervention is introduced and its effect measured; however, there is no random assignment of subjects.

r. The correlation coefficient; also called Pearson's *r;*

R^2. The coefficient of multiple determination; the proportion of variation in a dependent variable that is explained by a set of independent variables.

r^2. The coefficient of determination; the proportion of variation in one variable that is explained by another; a more precise measure of correlation between two variables.

random sample. A sample selected from a population in such a manner that each subject has an equal probability of being selected.

randomization. The process by which subjects are allocated to two or more groups by chance; groups formed by randomization are likely to be equivalent to one another.

randomized controlled trial. An experimental design with randomization of subjects to groups and a control group.

range. The numerical distance between the highest and lowest values in a set of data; results from subtracting the lowest value from the highest value in a group of data; the simplest measure of dispersion or variability.

raw data. Data that have not been manipulated using statistical techniques.

RCT. Randomized Clinical Trial.

regression. See ordinary least squares regression, regression or logistic regression.

regression coefficient. Beta; represents the change in dependent variable that accompanies a one-point increase in the independent variable.

reliability. The tendency of a test to result in the same score across multiple administrations; repeatability or reproducibility; the upper bounds of validity.

resources. Variously used to refer to factors of production, inputs or produced goods.

retest reliability. A form of estimating the reliability of measurements by administering the same test to the same group of people on two occasions, and then measuring the correlation between the scores.

retrospective. A study characterized by using data that have been collected prior to beginning the study.

risk-benefit analysis. A limited form of cost-benefit analysis that examines the benefits and risks of a particular procedure or alternative procedures.

robustness. The extent to which a service development is likely to prove efficient (e.g. through being flexible) even if parameters change. It is one desideratum by which options may be ranked. Whereas sensitivity analysis examines the sensitivity of the conclusions of an appraisal to variations in assumptions, robustness is a measure of the flexibility of an option in a changing world.

sample. A portion of a population of interest; used to draw inferences to the population.

sampling error. The differences between the sample and the population that occur due to chance and are not due to any systematic bias.

scale. A composite measure based on discrete items that measure the same construct; comprising a series of statements, questions, or words that, when scored in unison, provide a summary measure of an attitude, belief, or feeling.

scatter diagram. A graphical display of observations used to describe the relationship between two variables.

scatterplot. See scatter diagram.

Scheffé test. A commonly used post hoc comparison technique; the most conservative of the post hoc comparisons.

secondary data. Data that have been statistically analyzed and are presented only in summary form.

selection bias. A threat to the internal validity of a study that arises when there is a difference between the subjects in one group and the subjects in another; a threat to external validity when the subjects who enter the study are not representative of the population.

sensitivity. The proportion of true positives that are labeled positive.

sensitivity analysis. An analytical process that examines how results change when the values of key variables are changed.

significance level. The probability of rejecting the null hypothesis when it is true; alpha.

significance test. Also called a statistical test of significance; involves performing a statistical procedure in order to decide whether the differences observed are large enough that they could not occur by chance alone.

skewed. A distribution that deviates from the normal distribution by having most values in the upper or lower ends of the distribution; a positively skewed distribution has a longer tail to the right, and a negatively skewed distribution has a longer tail to the left.

social cost or benefit. Social costs (or benefits) are the sum of private and external costs (or benefits). Social costs (or benefits) include private costs (or benefits) together with any other effects that may create costs (or benefits) for other members of the community. Social costs are all opportunity costs. Thus the social cost of a medical procedure will include its effects on households and other sectors and not just the costs that are private to a hospital or clinic.

socioeconomic evaluation. A group of methods that provides information about the costs and consequences of medical products and services; used to identify which of several alternatives requires the fewest resources per unit output or produces the most output for given resources.

Spearman's coefficient of correlation. A statistic that describes the interrelationship of two categorical (ranked) variables; can range from 0 (no relationship) to +1 (perfect positive relationship) or −1 (perfect negative or inverse relationship); also called Spearman's rho.

specificity. The proportion of true negatives that are labeled negative.

split half reliability. A form of estimating the reliability of a scale by randomly dividing the scale into two halves and measuring the correlation between the two halves.

standard deviation. A measure of the variability or "spread" of a distribution; the square root of the variance.

standard error (of the estimate). In linear regression, a measure of the variability of the observed values of Y from the predicted values of Y; a small number indicates that the regression line fits the data closely.

standard error (of the mean). A measure of the sampling error; the standard deviation of all possible sample means around the population mean.

statistic. A measurable characteristic of a sample; contrast with parameter.

step-wise regression. A linear regression technique in which each independent variable is entered into the regression equation separately according to its strength as a predictor of Y.

study design. The structure of the research project; includes safeguards built into sample selection and data collection that enable the researcher to address the research hypothesis and to control for extraneous effects or competing hypotheses.

t-distribution. A bell-shaped and symmetrical distribution, but with the center of the distribution more spread out than the z-distribution; there stet families of t-distributions, each having a different shape according to the degrees of freedom in the test; used when the variance of the population is unknown and the sample size is less than 30.

time series analysis. A quasi-experimental design that employs data collected over several points in time; used when attempting to establish a causal relationship but an experimental study is not feasible.

transfer payment. A transfer of purchasing power from one group (for example, taxpayers) to another (for example, social security beneficiaries). Not to be confused with opportunity cost since transfer payments do not measure the most highly valued alternative use of resources, human or non-human.

treatment. An intervention introduced into an experiment; in ANOVA, the groups that form the basis of analysis.

t-test. A test of statistical significance that tests whether two means are significantly different; based on the t-distribution; also called Student's t-test.

true negative. A case that is accurately identified as being healthy.

true positive. A case that is accurately identified as having disease.

two-tailed hypothesis. A research (or alternative) hypothesis that only states there will be a difference between two groups, but does not specify the direction of the difference.

two-way ANOVA. An ANOVA that compares groups on the basis of two independent variables; see analysis of variance.

type I error. The error of rejecting the null hypothesis when it is true; stating that there was a significant effect or difference when in reality there is none.

type II error. The error of accepting the null hypothesis when it is false; stating that there was no significant effect or difference when in reality there is.

uncertainty. Usually applied to future events, costs and benefits. Sometimes attempts to "quantify" it are made by assigning probabilities based on past experience or derived by judgments of various kinds. Sometimes alternative scenarios of the future are devised. Out of the infinity of possible futures, the art lies in trying to narrow down the range to a manageable set of imaginable possibilities that, between them, encompass what are seen as the main characteristics of these possibilities.

utility. The value assigned to an outcome.

utility analysis. A method of measuring health outcomes in terms of the preferences that individuals express for being in particular health states; provides a common unit in order to compare different types of outcomes.

utilization. The intensity of use of medical resources per period. Overutilization is use in excess of some stipulated (etc.) rate: the bench-mark implied varies from context to context and the reader should be alert to its ambiguity.

validity. The tendency of a test to measure reality accurately; accuracy; how closely data conform to reality.

value. In economics usually taken as the maximum amount that an individual or group is willing to pay for a particular benefit. Marginal value is the value of marginal benefit: the maximum amount individuals are willing to pay for an increment of benefit.

value judgment. An ethical opinion made either implicitly or explicitly that a particular course of action, institutional arrangement, and so on ought to be implemented, or is itself good. For example, the judgment that consumers' willingness to pay ought to determine the allocation of health care services is a value judgment. The judgment that the location and type of services actually provided is determined by willingness to pay is not a value judgment. Economic appraisals typically involve many kinds of judgment, only some of which are judgments of value.

value of life. Reduced mortality/increased life-expectancy is a common benefit of health programs whose appraisal will sometimes require a value to be placed on such benefits. There are broadly three approaches. The human capital approach assesses the value as the present value of expected future earnings. This has been widely discredited for its partial nature and because of the discrimination it implies against the very young, the old, females, chronic sick, etc. The social decisions approach infers values from decisions made in the public sector: for example if a program to introduce childproof bottle caps for drugs at a cost of $50 per expected life saved is not adopted, then it is inferred that the average value of life for children at risk was not greater than $50. Its advantage is mainly in exposing the apparent inconsistencies in public decision making. The third approach enquires experimentally about the value placed by individuals on reductions in the size of the risk of death they confront with respect to any particular hazard. This approach is most consistent with the economic concept of efficiency.

variability. See variance.

variable cost. Costs that vary with the volume of services rendered.

variance. A measure of the variability or "spread" of a distribution.

willingness to pay. A method of valuing indirect costs based on the values people place on health and illness; based on valuing reductions in risk of illness or death.

within groups. In analysis of variance, that portion of the variance that is attributable to random differences between subjects within each group; see between groups; also called within column variance.

z-score. The standardized value that corresponds to the area between the value of interest and the mean; based on the *z*-distribution.

References

Akehurst RL, Buxton MJ (1985) Option appraisal in the NHS: a guide to better decision-making. Nuffield Provincial Hospitals Trust, London (Nuffield/York folio 8)

Arevalo JA, Washington AE (1988) Cost-effectiveness of prenatal screening and immunization for hepatitis B virus. JAMA 259(3):365–369

Barnum HN (1986) Cost savings from alternative treatments for tuberculosis. Soc Sci Med 23:847–850

Beck RT, Pauker SG (1983) The Markov process in medical prognosis. Med Decis Making 3:419–458

Bergner MB, Bobbitt RA, Carter WB, Gilson BS (1987) The sickness impact profile: development and final revision of a health status measure. Med Care 19:787

Bombardier C, Ware J, Russell IL, et al. (1986) Auranofin therapy and quality of life in patients with rheumatoid arthritis: results of a multicenter trial. Am J Med 81(4):565–578

Boyle MH, Torrance GW, Sinclair JC, Horwood SP (1983) Economic evaluation of neonatal intensive care of very-low-birthweight infants. N Engl J Med 308:1330–1337

Brook RH, Ware JE, Davies-Avery A, et al. (1979) Overview of adult health status measures fielded in Rand's Health Insurance Study. Med Care [Suppl] 17:1–131

Bush JW (1984) General Health Policy Model/Quality of Well-Being (QWB) Scale. In: Wenger NK, Mattson ME, Furberg CD, Elinson J (eds) Assessment of quality of life in clinical trials of cardiovascular therapies

Campbell DT, Stanley JC (1963) Experimental and quasi-experimental design for research. Mifflin, Boston

Chambers LW (1988) The McMaster Health Index Questionnaire: an update. In: Walker SR, Rosser RM (eds) Quality of life: assessment and application. MTP Press, Lancaster

Churchill DN, Lemon BC, Torrance GW (1984) A cost-effectiveness analysis of continuous ambulatory peritoneal dialysis and hospital hemodialysis. Med Decis Making 4:489–500

Crane VS (1988) Economic aspects of clinical decision making: applications of clinical decision analysis. Am J Hosp Pharm 45:548–553

Croog SH, Levine S, Testa MA, et al. (1986) The effects of antihypertensive therapy on the quality of life. N Engl J Med 314(26):1657–1664

Dahms WT, Molitch ME, Bray GA, et al. (1978) Treatment of obesity: cost-benefit assessment of behavioral therapy, placebo and two anorectic drugs. Am J Clin Nutr 31:774–778

Dao TD (1985) Cost-benefit and cost-effectiveness analysis of drug therapy. Am J Hosp Pharm 42:791–802

Doubilet P, Begg CB, Weinstein MC, Braun P, McNeil BJ (1985) Probabilistic sensitivity analysis using Monte Carlo simulation: a practical approach. Med Decis Making 5:157–177

Drummond MF, Stoddart GL, Torrance GW (1987) Methods for the economic evaluation of health care programmes. Oxford Medical, Oxford

Drummond MF, Teeling Smith G, Wells G (1988) Economic evaluation in the development of medicines. Office of Health Economics, London:1–36

Eisenberg JM, Kitz DS (1986) Savings from outpatient antibiotic therapy for osteomyelitis: economic analysis of a therapeutic strategy. JAMA 255(12):1584–1588

Eisenberg JM, Koffer H, Finkler SA (1984) Economic analysis of a new drug: potential savings in hospital operating costs from the use of a once-daily regimen of a parenteral cephalosporin. Rev Infect Dis [Suppl 4] 6:S909–S923

Eisenberg JM, et al. (1987) What is the cost of nephrotoxicity associated with aminoglycosides? Ann Intern Med 107:900–909
Evans RW, Manninen DL, Overcast TD, et al. (1984) The national heart transplantation study: final report. Battelle Human Affairs Research Centers, Seattle
Fleiss JL (1981) Statistical methods for rates and proportions. Wiley, New York
Geweke J, Weisbrod BA (1982) Clinical evaluation vs. economic evaluation: the case of a new drug. Med Care 2(8):821–830
Hartunian NS, Smart CN, Thompson MS (1980) The incidence and economic costs of cancer, motor vehicle injuries, coronary heart disease, and stroke: a comparative analysis. Am J Public Health 70:1249–1260
Henriksson P, Edhag O (1987) Cost-effectiveness comparison of estrogen therapy and orchidectomy in patients with prostatic cancer. Int J Technol Assessm Health Care 3:523–529
Hinman AR, Koplan JP (1984) Pertussis and pertussis vaccine. JAMA 251(23):3109–3113
Huck SW, Cormier WH, Bounds WG (1974) Reading statistics and research
Huse DM, Oster G, Weisbrod BA, et al. (1988) The cost-effectiveness of transdermal nitroglycerin in the Michigan medicaid program: a preliminary report. In: van Eimeren W, Horisberger B (eds) Socioeconomic evaluation of drug therapy. Springer, Berlin Heidelberg New York
Jachuk JS, et al. (1982) The effect of hypotensive drugs on the quality of life. J R Coll Gen Pract 32:103–105
Jonsson B (1983) Diabetes – the cost of illness and the cost of control. Acta Med Scand [Suppl] 671:19–27
Kaplan RM, Hartwell SL, Wilson DK, Wallace JP (1987) Effects of diet and exercise interventions on control and quality of life in non-insulin-dependent diabetes mellitus. J Gen Intern Med 2:220–228
Kassirer JP, Moskowitz AJ, Joseph L, Pauker SG (1987) Decision analysis: progress report. Ann Intern Med 106:275–291
Katz S (ed) (1987) The Portugal Conference: measuring quality of life and functional status in clinical epidemiological research. J Chronic Dis 40:459–650
Kinosian BP, Eisenberg JM (1988) Cutting into cholesterol; cost-effective alternatives for treating hypercholesterolemia. JAMA 259(15):2249–2254
Koplan JP, et al. (1979) Pertussis vaccine – an analysis of benefits, risks and costs. N Engl J Med 301:906–911
Levin RI (1981) Statistics for management. Prentice-Hall, Englewood Cliffs
Levine S, Croog SH (1984) What constitutes quality of life? A conceptualization of the dimensions of life quality in healthy populations and patients with cardiovascular disease. In: Wenger NK, Mattson ME, Furberg CD, Elinson J (eds) Assessment of quality of life in clinical trials of cardiovascular therapies. Le Jacq, New York, pp 46–58
Lohr KN, Ware JE (eds) (1987) Proceedings of the advances in health assessment conference. Palm Springs, California 19–21 February 1986. J Chronic Dis 40:1S–191S
Lohr KN (ed) (1989) Advances in health status assessment: Conference proceedings. Med Care [suppl.] 21:S1–S294
Lubeck DP, Spitz PW, Fries JF, et al. (1986) A multicenter study of annual health service utilization and costs in rheumatoid arthritis. Arthritis rheum 29(4):488–493
Luce BR, Schweitzer SO (1978) Smoking and alcohol abuse: a comparison of their economic consequences. N Engl J Med 298(10):569–571
Luce BR, Weschler JM, Underwood C (1989) The use of quality of life measures in the private sector. In: Mosteller F, Falotico-Taylor J (eds) Quality of life and technology assessment. National Academy Press, Washington DC
McDowell I, Newell C (1987) Measuring health: a guide to rating scales and questionnaires. Oxford University Press, New York
McNeil BJ, Pauker SG (1984) Decision analysis for public health: principles and illustrations. Annu Rev Public Health 5:135–161
McNeil BJ, Weichselbaum R, Pauker SG (1981) Speech and survival: trade-offs between quality and quantity of life in laryngeal cancer. N Engl J Med 305:982–987

Mulley AG, Silverstein MD, Dienstag JL (1982) Indications for the use of hepatitis B vaccine, based on cost-effectiveness analysis. N Engl J Med 1:644–652

Najman JM, Levine S (1981) Evaluating the impact of medical care and technologies on the quality: a review and critique. Soc Sci Med 15:107–155

Neuhauser D, Lewicki A (1975) What do we gain from the sixth stool guiac? N Engl J Med 293:226

Norrby SR, Eriksson M, Ottosson E (1986) Imipenem/cilastatin versus gentamicin/clindamycin: a cost-effectiveness study. Scand J Infect Dis 18:371–374

Oster G, Epstein AM (1987) Cost-effectiveness of antihyperlipemic therapy in the prevention of coronary heart disease. JAMA 258:2381–2387

Oster G, Colditz GA, Kelly NL (1984) The economic costs of smoking and benefits of quitting for individual smokers. Prev Med 13:377–389

Pauker SG (1976) Coronary artery surgery: the use of decision analysis. Ann Intern Med 85:8–18

Pauker SG, Kassirer JP (1978) Clinical application of decision analysis: a detailed illustration. Semin Nucl Med 8:324–335

Pauker SG, Kassirer JP (1987) Decision analysis. N Engl J Med 316:250–258

Pliskin JS, Shepard DS, Weinstein MC (1980) Utility functions for life years and health status. Operat Res 28:206–224

Radloff LS (1977) The CES-D scale: a selfreport depression scale for research in the general population. Appl Psychol Measurem 1:385–401

Revicki DA, Underwood C (1988) Quality of life and non-insulin dependent diabetes mellitus. Battelle Human Affairs Research Centers, Washington

Roland M, Morris R (1983) A study of the natural history of back pain: development of a reliable and sensitive measure of disability in low-back pain. Spine 8:141–144

Sackett DL, Snow JC (1979) The magnitude of compliance and noncompliance. In: Haynes BR, Taylor DW, Sackett DL (eds) Compliance in health care. Johns Hopkins University Press, Baltimore, pp 11–22

Sackett DL, Torrance GW (1978) The utility of different health states as perceived by the general public. J Chronic Dis 31:697–704

Sasaki A, Eisenberg JM (1987) Cost-effectiveness analysis of treatment for esophageal varices in Japan. Int J Technol Assessm Health Care 3:575–586

Schoenbaum SC, et al. (1976a) The swine-influenza decision. N Engl J Med 295:759–765

Schoenbaum SC, Hyde JN, Bartoshesky L, Crampton K (1976b) Benefit-cost analysis of rubella vaccination policy. N Engl J Med 294(6):306–310

Shapiro M, Schoenbaum SC, Tager IB, Munoz A, Polk F (1983) Benefit-cost analysis of antimicrobial prophylaxis in abdominal and vaginal hysterectomy. JAMA 249:1290–1294

Simon DG (1986) A cost-effectiveness analysis of cyclosporine in cadaveric kidney transplantation. Med Decis Making 6:199–205

Snider DE, Caras GJ, Koplan JP (1986) Preventive therapy with isoniazid; cost-effectiveness of different durations of therapy. JAMA 255(12):1579–1583

Sox HC et al. (1988) Medical decision making. Boston, Butterworth

Stewart AL, Hays RD, Ware JE (1988) The MOS Short-Form General Health Survey: reliability and validity in a patient population. Med Care 26:724–735

Thompson MS, Read JL, Hutchings HC, Paterson M, Harris ED (1988) Cost-effectiveness of Auranofin: results of a randomized clinical trial. J Rheumatol 15:35–42

Tompkins RK, Burns DC, Cable WE (1977) An analysis of cost-effectiveness of pharyngitis management and acute rheumatic fever prevention. Ann Intern Med 86:481–492

Torrance GW (1986) Measurement of health state utilities for economic appraisal. J Health Econ 5:1–30

Torrance GW (1987) Utility approach to measuring health-related quality of life. J Chronic Dis 40(6):593–600

Von Neumann J, Morgenstern O (1953) Theory of games and economic behavior. Wiley, New York

Walker SR, Rosser RM (eds) (1988) Quality of life: assessment and application. MTP Press, Lancaster

Washington AE, Browner WS, Korenbrot CC (1987) Cost effectiveness of combined treatment for endocervical gonorrhea. Considering co-infection with Chlamydia trachomatis. JAMA 257:2056–2060

Weinstein MC (1980) Estrogen use in postmenopausal women – costs, risks, and benefits. N Engl J Med 303(6):308–316

Weinstein MC, et al. (1986) Cost-effectiveness choice of antimicrobial therapy for serious infections. J Gen Intern Med 1:351–363

Weisbrod BA, Test MA, Stein LI (1980) Alternatives to mental hospital treatment. II. Economic benefit-cost analysis. Arch Gen Psychiatry 37:400–405

Weiss JC, Melman ST (1988) Cost-effectiveness in the choice of antibiotics for the initial treatment of otitis media in children; a decision analysis approach. Pediatr Infect Dis J 7:23–26

Wenger NK, Mattson ME, Furberg CD, Elinson J (eds) (1984) Assessment of quality of life in clinical trials of cardiovascular therapies. Le Jacq, New York

Wennberg JE, Freeman JL, Culp WJ (1987) Are hospital services rationed in New Haven or over-utilized in Boston? Lancet 1:1185–1189

Wernli J, Sproll T (1988) Sozio-ökonomische Bewertung von neuen Arzneimitteln. Pharm Ind 50:304–307

Willems JS, et al. (1980) Cost-effectiveness of vaccination against pneumococcal pneumonia. N Engl J Med 303:553–559

Wodinsky HB, DeAngelis C, Rusthoven JJ, Kerr IG, Sutherland D, Iscoe N, Buckman R, Kornijenko M (1987) Re-evaluating the cost of outpatient cancer chemotherapy. Can Med Assoc J 137:903–906

Postscript: Successful Socioeconomic Evaluation of Health Care Services

B. HORISBERGER

Yourself must feel it first, your end to capture.
Unless from out the soul it well,
And with a fresh, resistless rapture
Your hearers' very hearts compel, –
But heart to heart ye will not sway and fashion,
Save in your heart ye feel it first
(Goethe in Faust, Part I, translated by A. G. Latham)

Of paramount importance to the acceptance of the results of a socioeconomic study is the intrinsic understanding of the problem or the question it is trying to answer. Progressing from result to action, one has not only to identify the interdependencies between an organization and its environment. Equally important are the intrinsic mechanisms that use energy, physical and intellectual work to produce improved health or waste.

Action Planning

The results of any good and appropriately conducted socioeconomic evaluation are worthless, unless the health care organization (e.g., the health care system) is prepared to adopt the information and transform it into better actions in order to improve the performance of the system and the quality of outcome. For this, the organizational design must be flexible to allow for modifications in existing behavior. Systems theory is a method of dealing with the complexities of human interaction and of man with the material and natural world. As noted by Helmer (1967), "future developments cannot be forecast in isolation. A comprehensive and interdisciplinary integrated analysis is mandatory, even if the subject of immediate interest is relatively narrow."

The beneficial "fallout" from the studies in the past suggests a less than complete success, partly because of the large complexity of health care problems, the limited time of (short-term) studies, and the small amount of funding for meaningful subsequent organizational management. Understanding the anatomy and physiology of the health service and health care organizations begins with the concept of viewing an organization (in the case of a health care delivery) as an *open system*. In the formulation of Donabedian (1980) such a system can be viewed as a quasi-sequence of "structure", "process" and "outcome."

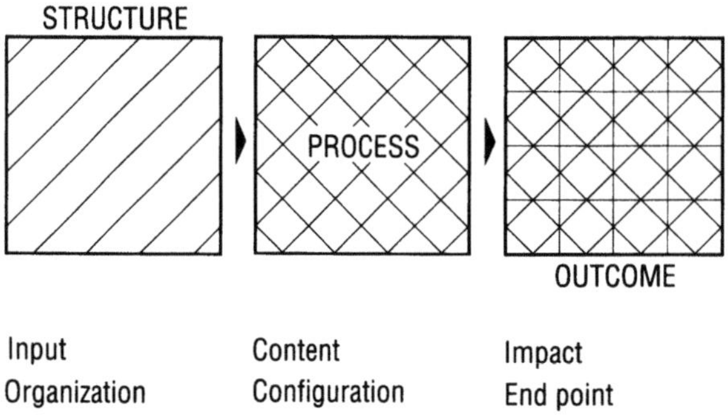

Fig. 1. The structure-process-outcome model (from Donabedian 1980)

By *structure* is meant the relatively stable charcteristics of the providers of care, of the tools and resources they have at their disposal, and of the physical and organizational settings in which they work. The study of structure as a means for assessing the quality of care is a rather blunt instrument, necessary but not sufficient. But a sufficiency of resources and a proper system design is necessary for protecting and promoting the quality of care.

The term *process* means the whole set of activities that go on within and between medical practitioners and patients. With regard to technical patient management (e.g., the performance of a diagnostic test or the prescription of a drug), the relationship between the characteristics of the process of care and its consequences is determined by the state of medical science and technology at any given time. The process quite often is the primary object of assessment. Alternative processes are analyzed and compared as to their merits. The basis for the judgement is what is known about the relationship between the characteristics of the medical care process and their consequences for the health and well-being of individuals and society.

The study of *outcomes* is an indirect approach to assess the quality of care "to mean a change in a patient's current and future health status, that can be attributed to antecedent health care" (Donabedian 1980). The validity of a specific element of process can be accepted only if a clear relationship to desirable outcomes has been established under adequately controlled conditions. But even when a decision to use outcome measures has been made, one must select which outcome should be measured and the source of data for assessment.

Structure, process and outcome are quite strongly interdependent at any time. In expanding Donabedian's trilogy of structure-process-outcome, we can adopt a more holistic understanding of health care and health service organizations, considering them as living societal organisms with their specific external and internal environment. To illustrate this view, Fig. 1 may be redesigned, integrating the overlapping influences between Donabedian's three components (Fig. 2).

Environment should be described at several levels, including the larger economic, political, and cultural context at the national level (e.g., industrialized countries, EEC, USA, Japan, Germany, Switzerland, etc.); or the configuration of the organization and personnel affecting the program (e.g., hospitals, health

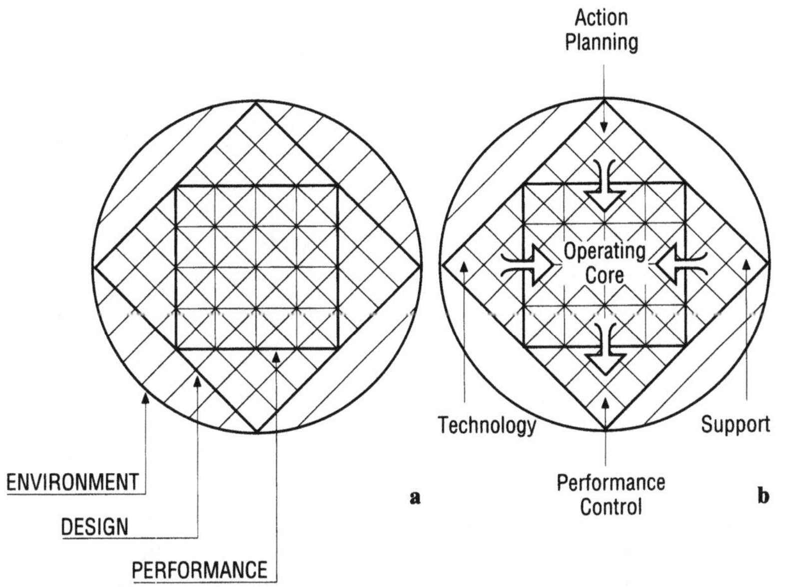

Fig. 2a, b The relation of **a** Donabedian's structure-process-outcome model to **b** the functioning of an organization

care centers, the immediate task environment, etc.); or resources directly involved in a specific program (e.g., care for elderly, mother and child care, treatment of hypertension, prevention of osteoporosis, etc.). *Design* in the narrower sense means services, procedures, and resources confined to the care of a specific illness; at the broadest it comprises all activities in the promotion of social, mental, and physical health, preventive measures, early diagnosis, care of illness, physical and social rehabilitation, etc. *Performance* can be viewed in terms of output quantities, use of resources per case or per disease group over time, provider satisfaction, patient satisfaction, relation between input or costs and output, relation between input or costs and outcome, quality of life aspects, etc. Although each of these three system components would merit a detailed examination, the purpose of this short description is to assess the principal organizational design component in order to understand where, when, for what, and under what circumstances the results of a socioeconomic analysis of the type described in this book can be successfully applied.

In order to understand the forces supporting or opposing the implementation of a new modality (on the basis or as a consequence of the foregoing approach), it seems useful to refer to the roles of the various actors in the health scene by referring to specific health service's organizations from the bottom up.

Outpatient Institution

At the simple level of organization of an outpatient institution, the individuals involved are expected to perform a set of related activities. For example, a physi-

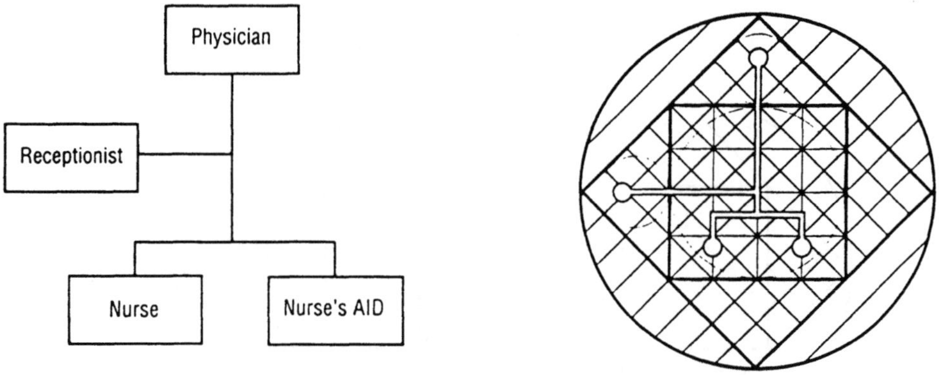

Fig. 3a, b Conventional model of **a** a simple outpatient organization (doctor's office) projected into **b** the environment-design-performance model

cian in his office measures the blood pressure in a hypertensive patient and decides to prescribe a new drug. The nurse is expected to dispense the medication. Subsequently, the physician monitors the care process and renews or continues prescription if he is satisfied with the result. A receptionist may be responsible for scheduling the patient's visits or fixing referral appointments at a cardiology clinic. She might also be responsible for performing laboratory tests or clinical tasks. Such a simple organization is illustrated in Fig. 3.

In a small institution like this simple outpatient organization, the suggestion for a systematic analysis seems perhaps superfluous or exaggerated. Individuals who perform a specific task can be readily identified. One has to deal with one or two persons if a new technology has to be implemented or tested. The simple process of informal communication and mutual adjustment needs no special consideration. However, to suppose that action planning or evaluating activities and controlling performance at this low level would be trivial is erroneous. The disadvantage of such simple structures is the lack of an independent adaptive subsystem that could be in charge of program adaptation, e.g., communicating with the project leader, answering questions of the work group involved in the production subsystem. No extra position is available for scheduling patients' visits; the receptionist has to take this extra charge. The critical areas in implementing a new technology need to be carefully identified. Regarding additional resources, one has obviously to deal with the head of the system (e.g., the practising physician), and this means additional time for planning first. Secondly, support is needed for the adaptive subsystem where no special position is available; this usually means information and training of the staff. Last but not least, the maintenance subsystem must be completed, and drugs and articles of consumption must be supplied. Owing to the relatively small number of patients treated in these institutions, any meaningful socioeconomic evaluation involves several institutions and coordination from outside, which must be conducted in a reserved manner, direct supervision is rarely possible. As an organization outgrows this simple state, informal regulations do not suffice and the coordination of subsystems has to be established. As an example, we can discuss the case of a small hospital.

Hospital Institution

In the setting of a hospital institution, the medical professionals are still the key figures but are typically in the position of the heads of a service or production subsystem. The people charged with overall responsibility for the organization, the "strategic apex", according to Mintzberg (1979), charged with ensuring that the hospital serve its mission in an effective way, are not involved in patient management. Many support units and technostructures are selfcontained. Positions within the structure are characterized by a larger corporate structure, which is superimposed on several smaller subunits, and possibly also by a high degree of vertical and horizontal differentiation and a great deal of stratification. In the illustrated example (Fig. 4), integration is highly formalized and represented by specific departments or positions that coordinate activities. In contrast to the simple structure in the free-standing physician's office, medical differentiation and technical specialization lead to multilevel management, and specialization of the production subsystems leads to horizontal differentiation. New subsystems are being found. The intrinsic characteristics of such a more complex design are revealed in Fig. 4.

A doctor's office or a small community health center consists of only a few elements and coordination is easy. However, looking at the functions of the different positions involved in a hospital, one can distinguish five distinct subsystems. The conventional model of this organization (Fig. 4a) presents only a static frame of this situation. In contrast, in the symbolic model (Fig. 4b), the operating core and the adjacent subsystems can be distinguished. According to Katz and Kahn (1966), the following are of importance:

- *Production subsystem* refers to work group activities that comprise the major technology function. It involves the recurring activities concerned with the dirrect provision of diagnosis and treatment.
- *Adaptive subsystem* refers to work group activities concerned with ensuring adaptation of the production subsystem to innovation and to internal or external loads.
- *Maintenance subsystem* refers to work group activities concerned with ensuring operational stability and high quality of infrastructures and logistics.
- *Managerial subsystem* refers to the work group activities concerned with coordinating and controlling the activities of the other subsystems, in particular also interactions with environment.
- *Performance control subsystem* refers to work group activities concerned with patient-related outcomes and physician-related or health practitioner-related outcomes.

Tension in the system results from built-in conflict as the system grows; this conflict arises between the suprasystem's need to control and the subsystem's attempts to retain a separate identity and autonomy. Successful implementation of innovation in such a system requires careful consideration concerning the distribution of competence on the managerial levels, and a thorough knowledge of the distribution of roles in the production subsystem. Strengthening the adaptive subsystem and adaptation of the maintenance subsystem (engineering department, pharmacy) needs careful consideration, too.

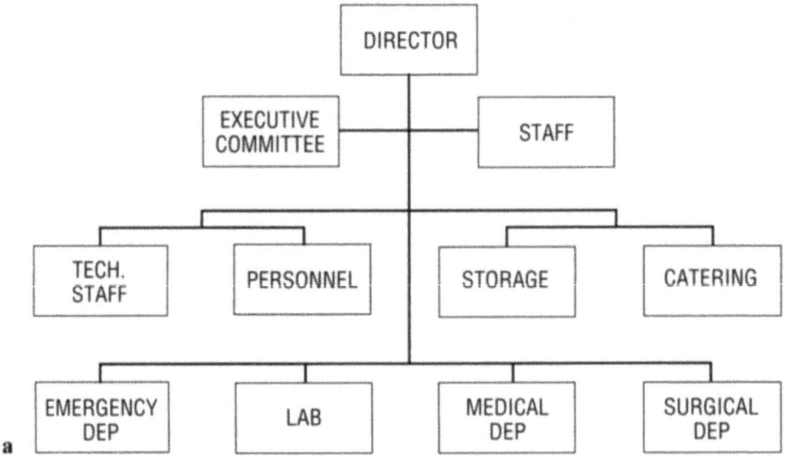

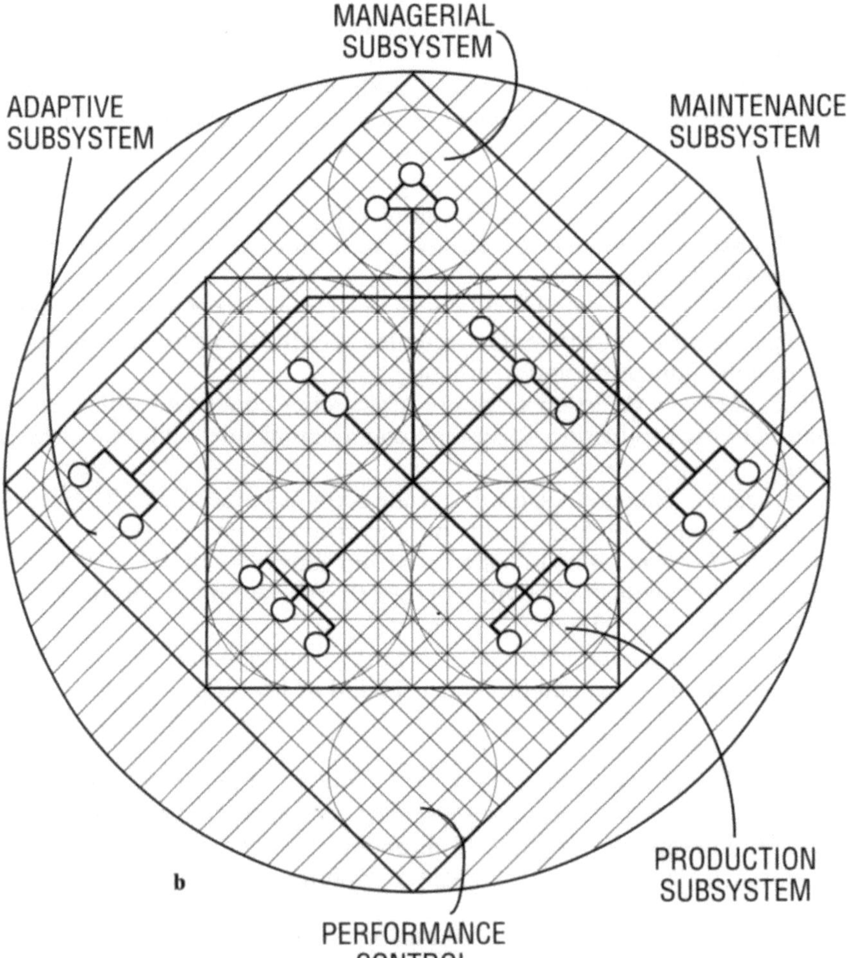

Fig. 4a, b Translation of **a** the highly formalized structure of a small hospital into **b** the functional environment-design-performance model

Undertaking a randomized clinical trial (RCT), the standard design for assessing health care interventions and other quasi-experimental designs must be evaluated by an ethics committee. This body examines the study from the patient's perspective. There may be two treatment groups, treatment and control (non-treatment), or more, such as various levels of treatment or various different therapies. Some problems are logistic rather than scientific.

Clinical trials at this operational level should be encouraged and should be organized so that "they can be afforded the best chance to be completed with meaningful results that could potentially influence policy. Evidence may not suffice – but it is a good start" (Balaban and Goldfarb 1983). Results can be especially useful and amenable to a study of cost-effectiveness if costs and expenditures are tracked concomitantly.

Networks

A regional or national health care delivery system is an extremely complex metastructure with different levels of decision and policy-making. At the apex, the political forces are predominant; at the hospital level, the medical professionals remain the key figures; at the outpatient or community level, professional structures besides doctors play an important role. There is a lot of competition between institutions, and the performance of the individual components may differ in efficiency and quality of outcome. Regional or nationwide arrangements in principle deal with two different types of settings, namely hospitals and organizations for ambulatory care. Since hospitals have been, in the past, the fastest growing segment in health care, hospital planning and hospital cost containment are firmly entrenched in national or regional health policy.

Such very complex organizations as a health care delivery network contain rather a high degree of uncertainty regarding the reaction to the implementation of innovation. On the other hand, they are quite stable as far as the overall architecture is concernd. A problem in planning socioeconomic evaluation at the national level or in a macroperspective is the emphasis on the need for financial resources. The application of one or two types of analysis is rarely sufficient; more often a network of evaluations will be required, as exemplified in Fig. 5.

Today most industrialized countries promote a reallocation of resources from hospital to primary care. The ideal option would be to stimulate primary care in independent outpatient settings and to decrease simultaneously hospital care and the complexities within hospitals. Unfortunately, this is not always achieved. Even when a new modality is successful in shifting treatment towards ambulatory care, the hospital structures are kept intact. From a theoretical point of view, the shift of medical care towards ambulatory settings should bring about a containment of hospital costs, however, in the real world the opposite takes place: some people and buildings get other functions, and hospital activities increase as well. At this degree of complexity, the experienced analyst will realize that implementing an innovation is a nonrational process and that the rational view resulting from a socioeconomic assessment of different health care technologies may be paralyzed by vested interests, political constraints, and the inertia of the system itself.

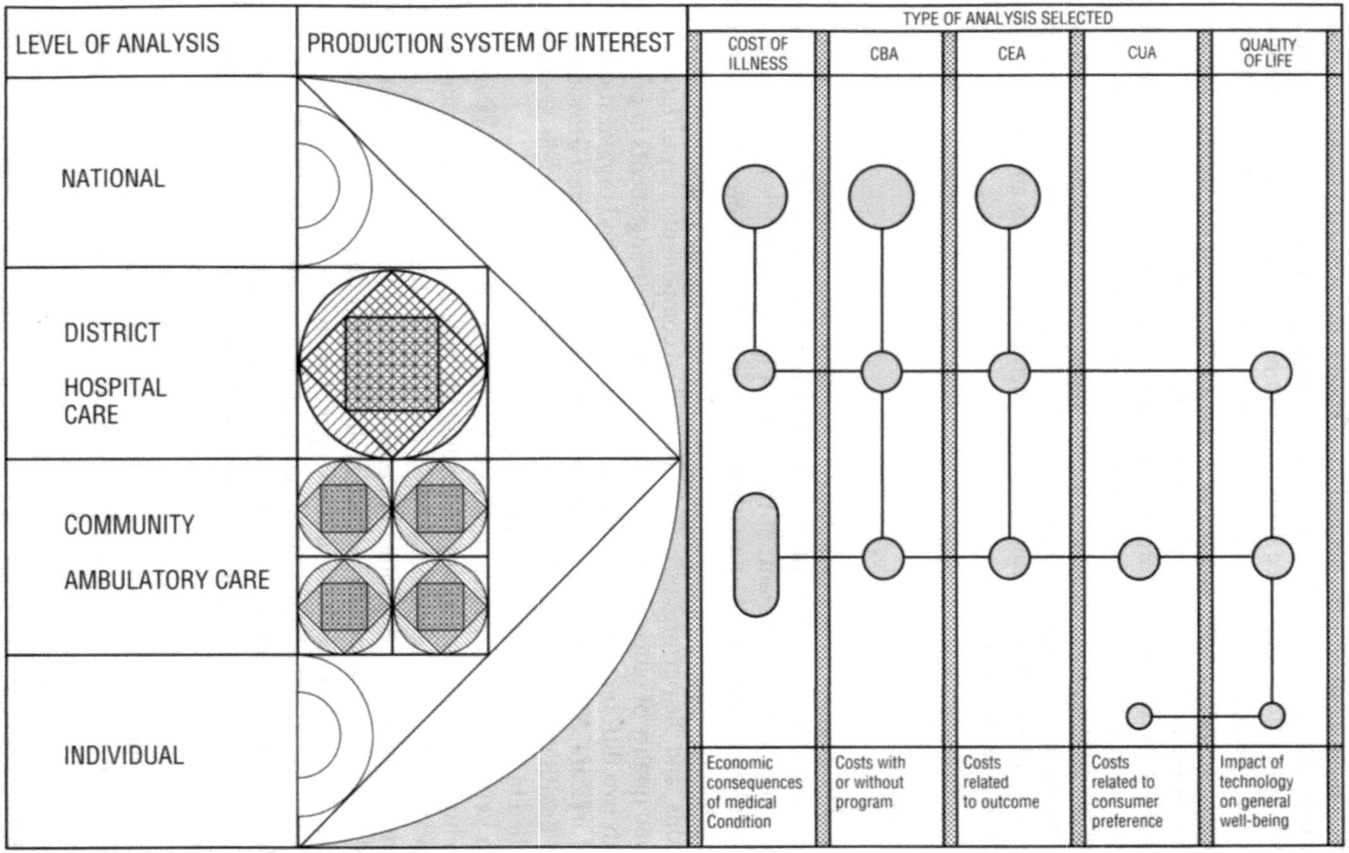

Fig. 5. The overall design of a health care system at the community, district, and national level, illustrating a network (or matrix) of different types of analyses combined to form an "economic dossier"

Research Synthesis

The so-called meta-analysis, or analysis of analyses, uses quantitative methods for combining or synthesizing the set of related socioeconomic studies. The synthesis can be used to draw conclusions about the effectiveness and safety of medical technologies including drugs. The increasing costs of randomized clinical trials, especially of surveys conducted to assess quality of life aspects, have generated interest in meta-analysis. This approach can determine effectiveness in a timely way without additional clinical trials when sufficient research already exists. One advantage of meta-analysis or pooling existing data over other techniques for research synthesis, such as group decisions, consensus methods, or simple literature review, is that this type of analysis focuses on the result of scientific evidence rather than on expert or peer opinion.

One major problem encountered in synthesis techniques lies in possible deficiencies in the original studies. Often, existing biases have to be adjusted or removed. Important details in design and statistical analysis have to be resolved before the results of different studies can be pooled. Often, the environment in which a specific study has been performed differs from the conditions prevailing in another situation or country. Often, the study has been conducted at another level. Microeconomic studies cannot be directly aggregated to the national level; they may refer to a specific selection of patients and conditions not representative for the entire population at risk, e.g., important elements of indirect costs may not have been considered.

Research synthesis per se is a formidable task and must start with a critical evaluation of the individual studies to be included in the synthesis. To this end the detailed description of the methods of evaluation explained in this manual will be of practical value.

Multidisciplinary Studies

Once we have reached the stage of multidisciplinary studies, it becomes clear that in performing socioeconomic evaluations of health services the conceptual skills of experts in medicine, the conceptual skills of sociologists, and the conceptual skills of economists are all complementary to one another. As we have stated elsewhere, multidisciplinary collaboration is the sine qua non of successful evaluation of the entire health care system as a productive social organization (Culyer and Horisberger 1983). This is not to say that the same is true at all levels of evaluation; indeed, there are types of evaluation that do not need multidisciplinary collaboration. What all types of studies require, however, is systems thinking, as illustrated in *Fig. 6.* Figure 6 shows a three-dimensional presentation of the interrelation between the level of analysis, the different types of analysis, and the different perspectives. The cube a shows on the left-hand side the organizational layers, from community and ambulatory care, through hospital care, and up to the aggregated systems level. On the right-hand side, the various types of socioeconomic analysis are presented. On the top face of the cube, the different perspectives, medical, social, and economic, are shown. The cube may be sliced according to

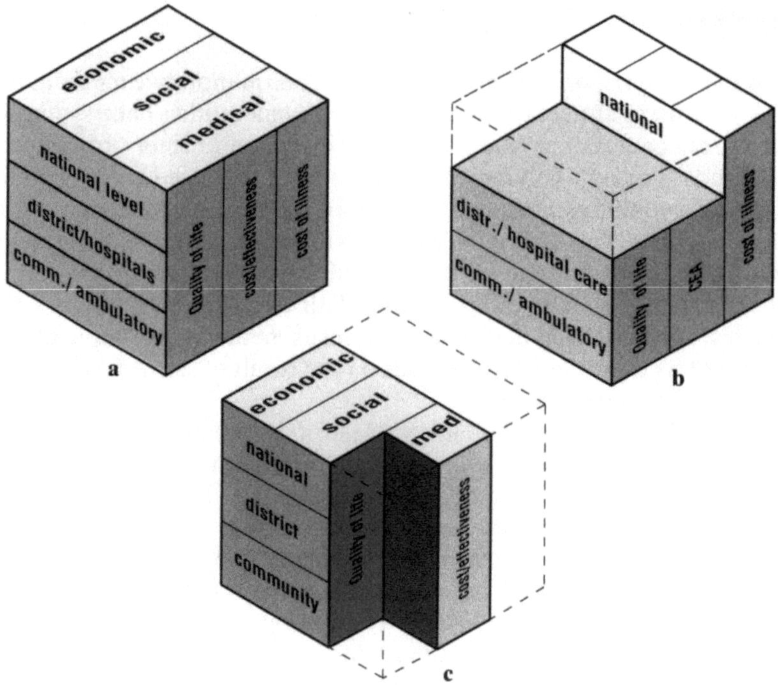

Fig. 6a–c Interrelation between the level of analysis, the different types of analysis, and the different perspectives

one's focus of interest. Cube b, for example, is sliced to assess the total costs of a specific disease in relation to medical interventions. In example c the cube is sliced from a socioeconomic perspective of one or more modalities and shows a set of factors that are relevant in that case.

Long-Term Technology Assessment

Once the effects of the short-term analysis of a new medical technology appear clear, additional or long-term analysis will be needed to ascertain and document the full effects of the technology (Bloom and Gessner 1989). Only then can the safety and efficacy of a modality be assured and its overall impact on health services be estimated. Since systems behavior and reactions might change from country to country and in any given country over time, meta-analyses and long-term technology assessment are important tasks to be fulfilled in oder to indicate the relative position of the major design of performance structure. By doing so, technology assessment can reduce the level of uncertainty and hence increase the probabiflity of optimizing the allocation of resources.

Research synthesis, then, has two dimensions; one is transorganizational and aims to assess the effects of a technology under different environmental conditions and settings, the other aims to evaluate expected outcomes over time. The latter aspect is especially relevant for research and development, since the lifecycle of a (new) technology is limited, and the quest for future innovations is a permanent challenge.

Health System Dynamics

An effective strategy for economic, social, and medical aspects of health care and health services development involves "finding the key log in the jam". Everybody knows that social systems undergo transformation in the course of time and that they will continue to change in the future, but each participant tends to exaggerate the risk of possible loss if change in the system works against his present interests, and people often refuse to acknowledge that there may be possible gains in the exchange. The methods presented and explained in this book can serve as instruments to expose both costs (or losses) and gains (or benefits) of alternative approaches to solving a given problem.

In order to apply input and output comparisons on a sound and standardized basis, the definition of the principal actors in the health care system helps to identify the driving forces in the system. They are identical in all systems in the different industrialized countries and there are five of them:

1. *The medical profession* will not remain as close to political power as it was in the 19th and at the beginning of the 20th centuries, but will still represent science and academia and take a defensive position with respect to the translation of medical values into monetary terms.
2. *The network of primary health care* will play an important role as an entry point to the health care system. The doctors themselves are the gatekeepers who welcome the individual patient, as the latter expresses a spontaneous demand by coming to see the doctor. The gatekeeper role fosters the idea that individual demand reflects medical need and that every citizen has the right to ask for all the services the specialized network can offer.
3. *The system of hospital care,* such as the primary care system, is still characterized by unlimited access opened by the professional expertise of the primary health sector or, in the absence of access to expert advice, is obliged to accept everybody in need upon self-referral.
4. *The insurance system,* implemented on political grounds in the late 19th century to enable the economically weak to obtain professional help without risking a financial catastrophe, has developed into a medical affluence, creating a carte blanche at everybody's expense, including the taxpayer's. Shortage of financial resources will influence future decisions and set a limit to unrestricted growth.
5. *Public opinion* is the fifth driving force in the system. The political battleground between the collective expression of individual interest and the economic constraint of a limited budget reflects not only a tense reality but brings forth vested interests. Public financing is translated into solidarity; unrestricted spending is advocated as a right to equity or equality.

In the struggle for an equilibrated welfare and health care system, a series of instruments are needed to adjust the balance between the myriad of demands on the one hand, and limited resources on the other. Painful decisions will have to be made. Although the five interest groups mentioned are essential components of the health care system, it has become evident that their interaction is difficult to predict. The individual or vested interests of the medical parties have often resulted in the quasi-autonomous development of medical areas. Medical doctors and hospital administrators tend to expand or consolidate their institutions in order to reach a higher peer status or social prestige, or to generate higher revenues. Through specialization and the rapid adoption of new technologies, they create new markets and attract new clients. Controlling this expansion is not easy. Most attempts, such as certificates of need, have not been very successful. In some countries, such as the United States, the certificates of need were undercut, e.g., by philanthropic donations. Once a new tool or machine has been placed in a private or public setting, the neighbouring institutions are forced to follow in order to offer equal access to all their patients. A lower remuneration of the individual medical act in a fee-for-system in Japan, in the Netherlands, or in Switzerland, did not discourage the medical doctor or the hospital, but resulted in a higher output to compensate for the loss of income to physicians.

The Assessor's Commitment

To grapple with such complexity, socioeconomic analysis, properly conducted, may be a valuable aid to the decision maker. However, economic rationality will rarely be sufficient in the decision making process. The ultimate decision in health care matters actually follows the rules of the game that are specific to the health system of each country. They comprise a set of norms regulating medical practice and jurisdiction, and are determinded by the behavior of doctors, the organization of health insurance, the media and so on. The incentive structure thus created can suppress both economic rationality and good medical practice.

Although the technical aspects of socioeconomic evaluation of medications can be described in scientifically defined analytic terms, the impact that economic studies of this type have on decision making depends on all shorts of value judgments expressed by many individuals in the overall socioeconomic system of a country. To take an extreme case: arming barefoot medical aides in the developing world with modern technology may be grossly less effective than arming them with the skills to persuade and help people to change harmful lifestyles. The same is often true in the developed world, and it applies not only to the technology in question, but also to other technologies with which it may be compared. The judicious selection of prima facie relevant alternatives, the effectiveness of which is to be compared, involves asking the relevant question in such a fashion as to allow for the effect of other influential factors, namely the availability of human resources.

The successful analyst must not only be familiar with the techniques of socioeconomic analysis, but also be willing to communicate with the various actors in the game (e.g., medical doctors, administrators, epidemiologists, patients, sociologists, etc.). In other words, he must be willing and ready to adopt a multidisciplinary approach. It can be fatal to rely on the hypothesis that the actors involved themselves accept the principle of economic efficiency. It would be safer to acknowledge the fact that in a social system every party tends to play the game with a particular interest in view. For instance, at the microlevel, one should be aware of the fact that the clinicians are in general more responsive to the argument of quality than to the one of economy, although the two aspects might express identical values but in different terms. Good quality in outcome might not guarantee an economic benefit, but poor quality is almost certainly a loss, at least to the patient. On the other hand, the higher cost of a procedure can be offset by a superior quality in outcome. This, however, has to be demonstrated.

This leads to still another field of interest to the socioeconomic evaluator. Especially in the assessment and appraisal of drug programs, the quality of a medication might be expressed in terms of efficacy and safety. With two products that are equally efficacious but different in costs (or price), it seems not only useful but mandatory to evaluate the risk/benefit relation and to communicate the nature and scale of this ratio to health professionals, regulatory agencies, and politicians in terms of human suffering and monetary value. Especially now that patients and consumer organizations have become more aware, the drug safety/risk aspect should be incorporated in any type of socioeconomic evaluation of drugs.

The design of an evaluative study and the appropriate specification of the cost and benefit elements depend crucially on the nature of the question that one is seeking to answer. One special problem is the organization of interdisciplinary cooperation in socioeconomic studies. A group needs to learn to work together, where one part knows a great deal about medicine and the other a great deal about economics, but there are only few individuals who are knowledgeable in both areas. The essential task, namely to convey the economic perspective to the physician and to transmit clinical knowledge to the economist/analyst, can only be achieved through sustained interaction in a working team. The medical practitioner and the economist might take different points of view on certain problems. To the physician and his patient it is, for instance, very important to know whether a particular therapy brings about a permanent relief or only a temporary postponement of the need for better but perhaps more dangerous or more costly therapy. To an economist that distinction is far less important. In the eyes of a physician, postponement can be viewed as a success (e.g., postponement of hospitalization, prolongation of life following palliative surgery) or as a failure (e.g., postponement of a definitive cure), because he argues at the individual level. To the economist this is different: to him postponement of a costlier intervention is a good thing, if this leads to a permanent reduction of the need for resources. Through a discounting process he can translate that saving into a present value and that is part of the benefit in the form of reduced expenditure. Costs are better incurred in the future than now, because the resources saved can be put to productive use in the meantime.

A word may be said here about the important aspect of indirect costs and benefits. The percentage shares of indirect costs attributable to the total disease costs are often much larger than the percentage shares of direct costs, e.g., the calculation of indirect costs presents some inherent difficulties in housewives and in elderly people. The widely used method of using work losses as a proxy of indirect costs may fall flat in the case of population subgroups not involved in the production process. Sick-leave compensation reflects social security regulation of disease and varies fairly substantially between one country and another. Apart from the question of the seriousness of complaints, differences in the social security systems of different countries will account for the number of medical certificates issued and the length of sick-leave the doctors prescribe. Once the short-term direct effects of a new medical technology appear clear, additional and long-term analyses seem necessary to assess the indirect effects. Unfortunately, this type of study is only infrequently performed. This often leads to incomplete understanding of the modality's medical, social, and economic impact.

Among the manifold criticisms of the instrument of socioeconomic evaluation a few might be cited:

- The specific sociodemographic and economic situation or the legislation of a country are not considered, and therefore results are poorly applicable to follow-up actions.
- The reports are often weak in practical knowledge of an existing design (in the broadest sense) of the given area.
- Some recommendations or conclusions are politically or professionally so naive as to be impracticable.
- There is too much emphasis on the technology or modality and not enough on social and institutional factors. Consideration is often given to the best possible use of a technology when in fact only average use is the reality.
- Studies are too broad in scope and tend towards generalization.
- The study fails to identify and analyze a meaningful set of alternative approaches and solutions.

Many of these items reflect the overestimation of the instrument of socioeconomic evaluation, which certainly has great merits, but also has limitations. Nevertheless, the successful implementation of the results of socioeconomic studies requires a comprehensive approach, a careful selection of the specific areas of application, an appropriate policy, and good planning. Once health planners or policy makers have defined the factors influencing the delivery or performance of health services in a specific field of interest, they must specify the scope and purpose of an innovation and indentify the criteria (productivity, efficacy, survival, quality of life, etc.). The aims of the study should be consistent with both the needs and resource limitations identified during the environmental assessment. The following topics need careful consideration:

1. Has a consensus been reached regarding the final goal of the analysis?
2. Is it clear why a study ought to be done?
3. Has the motivation and cooperation of all the actors involved been assured?
4. Who are the customers of a specific study, academics or policy makers?
5. Who is in a position to carry out the study, to whom should one go to get the study done, who are the experts in the field?
6. What are the criteria one should apply in assessing whether a research protocol is a good one?
7. How complete and thorough need the study be and how much time and money is available?

Finally a remark on the impact of socioeconomic analysis on policy making. In the past the success of socioeconomic assessment studies on long-term or even day-to-day decision making at the national or regional levels has often been disappointing. One reason might be the time factor. Policy makers often need information or advice in a very short time, such that the results of special studies are probably not available within the time accorded to the analyst. It may also be that the technical rationality of the alternatives offered for decision through the use of those instruments do not coincide with the political rationality of the power structures that regulate the allocation of resources in the health sector. More often, however, the analyst does not get involved at all in the decision making process, due to lack of interest or money, or both. In the long run, to serve the cause of good evaluation means to involve the health authorities and the regulating bodies alongside the socioeconomic evaluator. Better data must be made accessible and must be made comprehensible to the public at large. Their implications for the decision making process must be demonstrated in order to stimulate the necessary credibility. Only then will we stimulate the incentives for more and appropriate (and only these) studies.

The reader of this book will be aware of the fact that no analysis or appraisal, no matter how sophisticated, will resolve problems. What it can do is to highlight them and identify more specifically what decision makers need to know, what the trade-offs are, what the likely pros and cons are. It is an aid to, not a substitute for, public and professional decision making. This volume provides an excellent contribution to the critical understanding of a report on an economic evaluation of medications, although it could not cover all the possible aspects involved in different types of studies. It needs to be complemented by the specific characteristics of a morbidity to be treated, by the inherent risk of the disease, and by the efficacy, safety, and risk of the different possible modalities under scrutiny. The strength of the manual lies in the systematic overview of the formal aspects of socioeconomic evaluations of health services. Examples of specific studies used throughout the manual to supplement the text help to clarify the issue. It meets the need for information at the clinical and the strategic level and avoids jargon. It offers a rich menu of principles and practice, useful to researchers in ambulatory and hospital settings, to policymakers and analysts at the level of third party payers, and health service planners.

Envoi

The coming decade will inevitably see much turbulence in the health sector of every country impelled by rising costs, shortages of resource staff, and the increasing demand from the public for ever wider access to fancier technologies. The medical profession, still strong in its collective organization, will encounter rising pressure from political parties and consumer movements which now jeopardize the profession's control of the health sector through collective bargaining over health care finance, insurance, and constraints and control by governmental authorities. Conflicting arguments about the contribution of individual and public responsibility will continue to challenge the traditional health care and social security systems. It will be crucial to the actors in the health arena to develop an independent and forward-looking attitude based on critical analysis and innovative speculation. Yet, in the end, the brave new world of future health care system will have to readjust the balance of collective contribution and individual demand to suit our human needs.

What emerges from all this? One simple lesson: a study that purports to be relevant must be tailored to the clients' needs. The "right" objective is not a question of principle, but of who the contractor or (imagined) client is. Since the interests of clients vary, a manual like this is not a substitute for individual decision making, but a valuable guide to good practice in the policy making process. The application of the presented tools of evaluation needs full insight into the conditions in which the health system operates in each country. Appropriate studies should be coupled with careful monitoring, so that the information generated could be used at a later decision point. If this volume supports such processes, then it will serve the immediate intention of the authors.

References

Balaban DJ, Goldfarb NJ (1983) Medical evaluation of health care technologies. In: Culyer AJ, Horisberger B (eds) Economic and medical evaluation of health care technologies. Springer, Berlin Heidelberg New York Tokyo, pp 16–31

Bloom O, Gessner U (1989) Long-term technology assessment. Intl. J. of Technology assessment in health care, 5, pp 215–226

Culyer AJ, Horisberger B (eds) (1983) Medical and economic evaluation: A postscript. In: Culyer AJ and Horisberger B (eds) Economic and medical evaluation of health care technologies. Springer, Berlin Heidelberg New York Tokyo, pp 347–358

Donabedian A (1980) The definition of quality and approaches to its assessment. In: Explorations in quality assessment and monitoring, vol. I. Health Administration Press, Ann Arbor, MI, pp 79–128

Helmer O (1967) Methodology of societal studies. The RAND Corporation, Santa Monica, CA, (Report no. P–3611)

Katz D, Kahn RL (1966) The social psychology of organizations. Wiley, New York

Mintzberg H (1979) The structuring of organizations. A synthesis of the research. Prentice-Hall, Englewood Cliffs, NJ

Curriculum Vitae of Authors

Anthony J. Culyer is a professor of economics and Head of the Department of Economics at the University of York, England. He has published widely in the economics of health and has held visiting professorships at universities in Australia, Canada and New Zealand. He co-edits the Journal of Health Economics.

Anne Elixhauser holds a Ph. D. in Health Services Research and has clinical experience as a physician assistant. She has performed cost-effectiveness analyses of computerized tomography, magnetic resonance imaging, diabetes, preconception care programs, and abatement of lead sources in paint and water. She is currently a research scientist with Battelle's Medical Technology and Policy Research Center. Her work has appeared or is expected in such journals as *International Journal of Technology Assessment in Health Care, Health Services Research, Medical Care,* and *Journal of Public Health Policy.*

Bryan R. Luce holds a Masters degree in Business Administration, a Masters of Science in Public Health, and a Ph. D. in Health Services Research with a specialization in health economics. He has extensive experience in cost-benefit and cost-effectiveness analysis as Senior Analyst with the Office of Technology Assessment, as Director of the Office of Research and Demonstrations for the Health Care Financing Administration, and currently as director of Battelle's Medical Technology and Policy Research Center. He is co-author of the textbook, *Cost-Benefit and Cost-Effectiveness Analysis in Health Care: Principles, Practice, and Potential* (Health Administration Press) and numerous articles appearing in such journals as *New England Journal of Medicine. American Journal of Public Health,* and *Journal of Community Health.*

Bruno Horisberger is an MD and was founder and first director of the Interdisciplinary Research Centre for Public Health in St. Gallen, Switzerland. He has published widely on the Socioeconomic evaluation of health care procedures, particularly with emphasis on their cultural and organisational contents. He is member of the editorial board of the International Journal of Health Sciences and co-editor of the book series on Health Systems Research by Springer-Verlag.

Subject Index*

absenteeism 69
action planning 163
Activities of Daily Living Scale 112
acupuncture 49
aging population 19
alpha value 129
alternatives 5, 49 ff, 61
analysis of variance 136
angina pectoris 63
angina 124
ANOVA 135, 136
antibiotics 38, 39, 44, 53, 86
arteriogram 118, 119, 120
arthritis 41, 49
auranofin 41
azathioprine 82

basic analytical techniques 134
Bayes' theorem 117
behavioral therapy 50, 51
benefits 59
– direct – 84
– indirect – 60, 84
– – opportunity cost approach 60
– intangible – 85
– negative – 59

beta-blocking drugs 50
brainstorming 4
budgetary analysis 42

cancer 50, 60, 79
cancer chemotherapy 48
captopril 112
cardiovascular diseases 63
Center for Epidemiologic Studies Depression Scale 112
central tendency 127
– measures of – 127
chance node 118
chi-square test 135, 138
– independent samples – 139
cholestipol 51
cholestyramine 46, 51
Cimetidine 34, 35, 47
clinical management
– pathways of 6, 44, 51, 54, 73
coefficient of determination 140
coefficient of multiple determination 143
combination therapy 53
comorbidities 86
compliance 74
confounders 86
consequences 68
– clinical – 68, 69
– determinants of 72
– economic – 69, 71
– gestalt of – 7
– health care resource utilization 70
– intangible – 75
– measurement of 83
– non-monetary – 72
– psychsocial – 69, 70
– types of 69
contingency table analysis 139
continuous peritoneal dialysis 124
control group 85
correlation analysis 140
cost containment 15
cost-benefit analysis (CBA) 2, 9, 32, 42, 73, 75, 94
– disadvantages 35
cost-effectiveness 74, 169
cost-effectiveness analysis (CEA) 3, 9, 37, 42, 74, 76, 95
cost-minimization analysis (CMA) 3, 32, 38, 43, 94
cost-of-illness (COI) studies 3, 32, 39, 43, 94
cost-shifting 24
cost-utility analysis (CUI) 35, 94, 124

* For further key-words please refer to Glossary p. 144–158

costs 8, 23
– alternative – 57
– assessment of – 56
– average – 63, 66
– direct – 8, 57 ff
– direct nonmedical – 58, 65
– discounted – 79
– economic – 24, 63
– financial (accounting) 24
– fixed – 8, 58, 59
– identifying – 62
– indirect – 8, 59, 65, 67, 84, 175
– – human capital approach 59
– intangible – 61, 65, 84
– marginal – 63, 66
– market value approach 59
– negative – 64
– nonmedical 8, 58
– opportunity – 8, 24, 57, 63, 66
– overhead – 63, 66
– postponed – 78
– proxy for – 63
– psychsocial – 59, 60, 65
– types of – 57, 64 ff
– variable – 8, 58, 59
cyclosporine cost-effectiveness 121
cyclosporine 82

decision analysis 117, 122
decision node 118
decision trees 53, 118, 121
decision-maker 4
decision-making 1, 6, 177
diabetes mellitus 40, 59
dialysis 82
discount rate 78
discounting 10, 28, 30, 77 ff
– consequences 78
dispersion 127

early discharge from hospital 48
economic dossier 170
effect size 132
efficiency 21
encephalitis 53
environment 164
epidemiology 22
esophageal varices 69
estrogen 64
estrogen therapy 50
evaluation, framework of 44
evaluator, socioeconomic 175
expected value 120
experimental group 85

F-test 137
factor 137
folding back 120

gambles 124
– standard – 125
General Health Rating Index 112 ff
glaucoma 50
gonorrhea 53, 54
goodness-of-fit 138

Hawthorne effect 91
health policy 169
health status 8
– changes of 21
health 52
– production of 52 ff
heart disease 60, 79
hemodialysis 124
hospital care 173
human capital approach 9
human capital 59, 60
hypertension 41, 127
hypertension treatment
– quality of life 73
hypothesis generation 22
hypothesis testing 128
– null hypothesis 128
– alternative hypothesis 128
hysterectomy 86

incidence 79, 80
independent variable 137
inferential statistics 127
inflation 77
insurance system 173

kidney transplantation 82, 121
Kruskal Wallis one-way ANOVA 135

laryngectomy 124
least square analysis 141
length of life 25
levels of measurement 134
– nominal, ordinal and interval data 134
long-term assessment 172

Mann-Whitney U test 135
marginal analysis 7, 26, 27, 28
marginal consequences 7, 8
marginal costs 7, 8
Markov processes 121
McMaster Health Index Questionnaire 112 ff
Medicaid 34, 35, 47
medical profession 173
Medicare 16
medications 17
– biomedical effects of 17
– efficacy 19
– safety 19
meta-analysis 171
methyldopa 112

modeling 91 ff
monetary values 62, 64, 70, 75
Monte Carlo simulation 121
morbidity 69
mortality 69
motor vehicle accidents 60
multidisciplinary studies 171
multiple regression 92
myocardial infarction 63

neonatal intensive care 124
network 169
– health care delivery – 169
– primary health care – 173
Nicotine Gum 37
nonparametric test 135
nonrandomized comparison group design 88
null hypothesis 137, 139, 140
nursing time 58

oat bran 51
one-group comparison 87
operationalization 92
opportunity cost 7
orchiectomy 50
ordinary least squares (OLS) regression 141
osteomyelitis 82
OTA 16
out-of-pocket payments 48
outcome 164
outpatient care 165 ff

P-value 129
parametric tests 135
Pearson product moment correlation 135, 140
penicillin 90
performance 165
perspective 73, 74
perspective costs 62
perspective 5, 45 ff, 61, 64, 72, 73
– of health care providers 48, 95
– of the patient 48, 75, 95
– of third party payers 47, 95
– societal – 45 ff, 62, 95
pharmaceutical industry 15
pharmacology 22
placebo 50
policy making 177
post hoc techniques 138
power 130
pre-test post-test design 87 ff
pregnancy 53
prevalence 79, 81
probability 117
– conditional – 117 ff
– posterior – 117 ff
– prior – 117 ff
process 164
productivity 59, 61, 67
productivity changes 21
propranolol 112
prospective data 11, 18
prospective studies 89
– types of 90
– parallel design 89
– time series 89
providers 16
Psychological General Well-Being Schedule 114, 115
public opinion 173

QESUNC 22
quality of life 9, 11, 25, 29, 40, 41, 69 ff, 109
– definition of – 109 ff
– measurement of – 112
quality of life (QOL) assessments 4, 32, 94, 109
quality of life scale items 113 ff
Quality of Well-Being Scale 112 ff
quality-adjusted life years (QALYs) 25, 36, 42, 70, 95, 124
quasi-experimental designs 89
questionnaires 96

RAD-AR VII
randomized clinical trial (RCT) 85 ff, 113, 169
– disadvantages of 87
randomized controlled experimental design 85
randomized controlled trial (RCT) 11
rating scale 125
ratios
– benefit-cost – 34, 64, 81
– cost-effectiveness – 37, 82
redistribution 24
regression 141
– hierarchical – 143
– linear – 141
– multiple – 141
– stepwise – 143
regression analysis 142
regression equation 142
renal failure 39
research question 4, 44, 72, 73
research synthesis 171
resource use 21
resources 62
retrospective studies 90
– disadvantages 91
– primary retrospective data 90
– secondary retrospective data 90
– types of – 90
rheumatic fever 90

sample size 130
scarcity of resources 24
scatter diagram 141
scatterplot 141
Scheffé-test 138
sclerotherapy 69
screening 50
sensitivity analysis 10, 11, 67, 75, 82 ff, 120 ff
– one-way – 121
– probabilistic – 121
Sickness Impact Profile 112 ff
smoking 81
socioeconomic analysis 174
– communication of – 174
– impact of on policy making 176
socioeconomic evaluations 2, 11
– choices 17
– compromises 17, 19, 31
– concepts 23
– consequences 2, 8, 25
– costs 2, 8
– disadvantages of – 176
– guide for evaluating 94
– history of 15
– incidence-based 79
– prevalence-based 79
– reason for performance 19
– types of 2, 84
socioeconomic hypotheses 5, 22
solidarity 173
spearman rank-order correlation 135, 140
standard deviation 127 ff
standard error of the estimate 142
statistical control 92
– primary – 92
statistical dependance 117
statistical significance 128
statistics 127
– central dentency 137
– normal distribution 127
stroke 60
structure 164
study design 11, 18, 83
– bims 85
– determinants of 84
– double-blind 85
– experimental 83
– observational 83
– prospective 83, 85
– retrospective 84, 90
subsystems 167
– adaptive – 167
– maintenance – 167
– managerial – 167
– performance control – 167
– production – 167
system dynamics 173
systems theory 163

t-test 135
technology assessments 172
– long term – 172
– short term – 172
technology 67
– rapidly changing – 67
tests
– one-tailed – 136
– two-tailed – 136
tetracycline 53
third-party payers 16
threshold analysis 81
time preference 10, 11, 77
time trade-off 125
time-motion studies 63
transfer payments 24, 67
transitional probabilities 121
transplantation 46
treatments 137
tuberculosis 57, 74
type I error 129, 136
type II error 129

US 16
– certificat of need 174
– Department of Defense 16
– Healt Care Financing Administration 16
– Office of Technology Assessment (OTA) 16
utilities 125
– methods for assessing 125
utility analysis 61, 70, 71, 75
utility 21, 69
utility values 71

vaccine
– hepatitis B 50, 72, 81
– pertussis 33, 44, 53, 81
– pneumococcal 36
– rubella 33
– swine-flu 69
validity 86
– external – 86
– internal – 86
valuation of resources 64
variance 127

willingness tp pay 60
willingness to pay method 9
within-patient design 87

Yates correction 140
years of life saved (YOLS) 25, 37

z-test 135

MIX
Papier aus verantwortungsvollen Quellen
Paper from responsible sources
FSC® C105338

If you have any concerns about our products,
you can contact us on
ProductSafety@springernature.com

In case Publisher is established outside the EU,
the EU authorized representative is:
Springer Nature Customer Service Center GmbH
Europaplatz 3, 69115 Heidelberg, Germany

Printed by Libri Plureos GmbH
in Hamburg, Germany